HYPOTHERMIA

Causes, Effects, Prevention

HYPOTHERMIA,

Causes, Effects, Prevention

Robert S. Pozos and David O. Born

NEW CENTURY PUBLISHERS, INC.

The author and publisher disclaim responsibility for any adverse effect resulting from the use of the information contained herein and strongly advise the reader to seek competent medical advice before undertaking any action that might produce a deleterious or otherwise undesirable result.

Copyright © 1982 by Robert S. Pozos and David O. Born
Cover design copyright © 1982 by New Century Publishers, Inc.

Printing Code
11   12   13   14   15   16

Library of Congress Cataloging in Publication Data

Pozos, Robert S.
  Hypothermia, causes, effects, prevention.

  Bibliography: p.
  Includes index.
  1. Hypothermia.   2. Cold—Physiological effect.
I. Born, David O.   II. Title.
RC88.5.P68   616.9′89   82-3519
ISBN 0-8329-0127-X   AACR2

In memory of
our fathers

Antonio S. Pozos
Jesse Woodruff Born

There are only two lasting bequests we can
hope to give our children. One of these is
roots; the other, wings.

Hodding Carter

Contents

Acknowledgments

The authors wish to acknowledge the support and assistance of Naida Yolen, Ph.D., Office of Sea Grant, National Oceanic and Atmospheric Administration, and Donald McNaught, Ph.D., Director of the Minnesota Sea Grant Program. Special appreciation is due to L.E. Witmers, M.D., Ph.D., and Edwin Haller, Ph.D., for their technical consultation and moral support. Roger Petry patiently led us through the mysteries of an invaluable word processing system, and the services of his assistants, Jane Fuller and Steve Sawyer, deserve far more praise than can be expressed here. Robert Hill, our editor at New Century Publishers, Inc., provided judicious advice when it was most needed and his firm belief in the importance of our subject matter was particularly encouraging.

We owe a great debt to the many scientists and physicians who studied hypothermia; while the efforts of many such people are recognized in our "Selected Readings" section, we wish to express our appreciation to all of them here as well.

We would be remiss if we did not bring to the public's attention the medical contributions made by the thousands of people who have fallen prey to hypothermia, by the dozens of volunteers who have subjected themselves willingly to the stresses of severe cold, and by the prisoners of Dachau, whose cold-induced deaths were an unconscionable travesty of scientific inquiry.

Last, we wish to acknowledge the unflagging support and good-natured indulgence of our wives and children — they more than anyone know the demands a book makes on its authors.

Robert S. Pozos
David O. Born

It is a psychological axiom that man will become so accustomed to dangers with which his daily life brings him in constant contact that he will not recognize them as dangers at all. While this is true, panic will strike him when he finds himself suddenly in positions infinitely less dangerous, but with which he is wholly unfamiliar and which he does not know instinctively how to combat.

HUNTING WITH THE ESKIMOS
Harry Whitney

HYPOTHERMIA

Causes, Effects, Prevention

CHAPTER 1

Cold: The Human Experience

Cold! Even the mention of the word can cause us to hunch our shoulders in a shiver. Whether it comes in the form of crisp, starry nights on the desert floor, the bone-racking cold of the North Sea, the subzero temperatures of a Minnesota blizzard or simply the incessant chill of old age, cold imposes itself on us like an unwanted, unrelenting visitor.

Stories about people suffering, or even dying from the cold bring to mind images of the great polar explorations or of those who lose their way during snowstorms. As for ourselves, actually suffering from severe cold seems like a pretty remote possibility. Because our technological society tends to isolate, or at least to shield us from our larger, natural environment, we are seduced into a false sense of security. We see ourselves as somehow "exempt" from the laws of nature. And then, when disaster strikes, we find ourselves unprepared and vulnerable.

Historically, severe winter storms have crippled many of our major cities, which are our centers of technology: the central plains, New York City and the entire eastern seaboard in 1888, Charleston, South Carolina in 1899 and 1973, Atlanta in 1973, Buffalo in 1957 and 1977, Boston and Chicago in 1977–78, and so on. In 1981 two successive storms hit the Twin Cities of Minneapolis and St. Paul.

Residents of Minnesota pride themselves on being able to handle the worst any winter can bring them, and one of their radio–TV stations boasts the world's largest private weather forecasting facility. In spite of all this, over 90,000 families were without power for 3–5 days, highways were blocked and communications were hampered. Among many whose lives and health were threatened were several hundred residents of a 20-story apartment building for the elderly. The building lost its heat and elevator services, and most of the occupants were unable to manage the long stairs. They could do nothing but sit and shiver while they waited for help from relief agencies.

Disasters provide our most dramatic encounters with the cold, but thermal stress on our bodies is an all-pervasive threat not limited to winter storms or polar expeditions: it's much more common than most of us realize.

There are many people, among them skiers, backpacking enthusiasts, off-shore oil rig workers, commercial fishing boat crews, scuba and deep-sea divers, hunters and soldiers, whose occupational or recreational pursuits expose them to chilling conditions which are obviously hazardous. There are many others, including the elderly, infants, winter travelers, children and the handicapped, who are exposed to less obvious, but equally perilous threats from the cold. None of us is immune.

Because severe heat loss can develop in so many ways, often attacking people in the safety of their own homes, the cold is a subtle, insidious danger that few of us understand completely. One reason is that we seldom stop to consider just how essential warmth is for survival. Every cell in the body requires warmth if it is to work properly. Too much heat, or too little, can cause damage to our cells. Every time the body's temperature drifts away from its optimal level (37°C or 98.6°F), the potential for a life-threatening breakdown exists.

When the body gains too much heat, we suffer sun stroke, heat exhaustion, fever, convulsions and even death. In contrast, if we lose too much heat, the bodily systems move slower and slower until they are scarcely functioning at all. Unless body warmth is restored *properly* and within a reasonable length of time, our life support systems will ultimately stop functioning and death will result.

Scientists and physicians use the term *hypothermia,* derived from the Greek *hypo* (under) and *thermia* (temperature), to describe a condition of the body when it is unable to maintain adequate warmth, and is operating therefore at subnormal *internal* temperatures. Hypothermia can develop very quickly: when a person is exposed to severe weather and lacks proper protection, the body can literally freeze to death in a matter of twenty or thirty minutes. Generally, it takes much longer. At other times, the development of hypothermia is so gradual that we don't realize what's happening until it's nearly too late.

An illustration of this point is the fact that hypothermia among the elderly is regarded as simply "natural" by many people. As a person ages, "everything seems to slow down;" everyone "knows" that older people "always feel a little cold." The truth is that older people don't *have* to feel cold. Many do, however, and the unrelenting cold to which they are exposed, even in their own homes, takes its toll on their health. We could easily avoid many hypothermia-related deaths that occur among the elderly each year if we were just more alert to hypothermia's warning signs.

Interestingly, one of the oldest written records of hypothermia deals with the elderly:

Now King David was old and advanced in years; and although they covered him with clothes, he could not get warm. Therefore his servants said to him, "Let a young maiden be sought for my lord the king and let her wait upon the king, and be his nurse; let her lie in your bosom that my lord the king may be warm." So they sought for a beautiful maiden throughout Israel, and found Abishag the Shunammite, and brought her to the king. The maiden was very beautiful; and she became the king's nurse; but the king knew her not.

(I Kings, 1–4)

This passage from the Old Testament is especially interesting not only because it deals with hypothermia, but because it also describes one of the standard techniques for rewarming the victim of hypothermia: body-to-body contact.

But king or commoner, coping with the cold has always been one of the greatest challenges faced by women and men. The cold is a mystical sorcerer, assuming whatever form might bedevil us the most: chilling drafts, drenching rains, frigid lakes, raging torrents, groaning ice packs or howling blizzards, to name but a few. Whatever the shape of the beast, our experience with the cold is seldom pleasant. However, if we are to understand hypothermia, we must learn how our minds and bodies respond to encounters with the cold.

Read, for example, how one twenty-four-year-old described a mid-winter Antarctic experience shortly after the turn of the century. There were days, he wrote, when it would

     . . . take you five minutes to lash up the door of the tent and five hours to get started in the morning . . .

     The trouble is sweat and breath . . . all this sweat instead of passing away through the porous wool of our clothing and gradually drying off us, froze and accumulated. It passed just away from our flesh and then became ice: we shook plenty of snow and ice down from inside our trousers every time we changed. . . .

     I got outside of the tent one morning. . . Once outside, I raised my head to look round and found I could not move it back. My clothing had frozen hard as I stood—perhaps fifteen seconds. For four hours I had to pull [a sledge] with my head stuck up, and from that time we all took care to bend down into pulling position before being frozen in.

     . . . For me it was a very bad night: a succession of shivering fits which I was quite unable to stop, and which took possession of my body for many minutes at a time until I thought my back would break . . . They talk of chattering teeth: but when your body chatters you may call yourself cold . . .

I for one had come to the point of suffering at which I did not really care if only I could die without much pain. They talk of the heroism of dying—they little know—it would be so easy to die, a dose of morphia, a friendly crevasse, and blissful sleep. The trouble is to go on.

THE WORST JOURNEY IN THE WORLD
Apsley Cherry-Garrard

The two-volume account of Cherry-Garrard's "worst journey" is a classic study in fatigue. His three-man party spent weeks dragging sledges across Antarctica on a scientific expedition. During those weeks *every second* involved a battle with subzero temperatures and high winds. They had not so much relief as a warm sleeping bag, for the severe cold turned their sleeping bags, like their clothes, into sheets of icy armor. Stress and fatigue wore the men down; the cold simply crushed them. It took an extraordinary effort just to *care* about survival, let alone to do something about it.

Fatigue, as we shall see, is hypothermia's doorstep. As the body's resources are depleted, there is no energy left to resist the cold; hypothermia steps in and begins its destructive processes.

Few of us will have to endure the stress of a mid-winter polar journey as young Cherry-Garrard did, but one doesn't have to be an explorer or an adventurer to suffer fatigue, which with fear and mild hypothermia, has been cited as the cause of a high school band "disaster" that occurred in the fall of 1981 at a football game time in Flint, Michigan. The temperature was 31°F (−.5°C), with a wind chill factor of 11°F (−12°C). A number of band members apparently were very tired, but nonetheless anxious to present their half-time show. First, one student became ill, then several others collapsed; panic spread, and before things were brought under control 32 young people were taken to nearby hospitals with symptoms which included shivering, hyperventilation and weak pulse rates, all classic signs of mild hypothermia.

A hospital spokesman commented that "a combination of cold and fatigue caused some [of the students] to have body stress and chills." One frightened boy said simply, "we didn't know what was wrong because everybody was falling down."

It was also fatigue which led to many of the 3,000 deaths experienced by Washington's army at Valley Forge in the winter of 1777–1778. The weather was foul, but not severe. The soldiers were exhausted by hurried marches, and morale was low. Hastily built shelters offered scant protection from the weather, which included frequent rain and snow. Malnutrition, inadequate clothing and prolonged exposure to the cold were all that was needed to set the stage for hypothermia.

While stories of severe cold and hypothermia often have a tragic ending (chiefly because the victims were uninformed about heat loss and survival techniques), there are accounts of cold-related incidents in which the mechanisms of the body's hypothermic response work in such a way as to ensure survival.

Such a story involves an eleven-year-old boy whose mother, noticing a sudden silence in the backyard, went to look for her son and was told by one of his playmates that he had fallen into the creek. Rushing to the creek, she saw his hat floating on the water. A rescue squad soon arrived and began searching the 48°F (8.8°C) water for the child. After a 15-minute search they found him, fully submerged.

His skin was blue, there was no pulse, and his pupils were dilated; there were no vital signs. Cardiopulmonary resuscitation was started immediately and continued during a 20-minute ride to the hospital. When the boy arrived at the emergency room, his rectal temperature was 93°F (33.8°C) (well below normal), and he showed no brain activity.

A medical team worked for six straight hours before they were able to notice any improvement in the boy's condition. It was not until nine hours after rescue that a strong eye pupil response could be detected. Two days later the boy sat up, coughed and began to play with the toys by his bed.

A similar experience befell a 25-year-old diver who was investigating a shipwreck 60 feet down in the Straits of Mackinac. While inside a dark room on the ship, the diver panicked and tried to escape through a porthole, breaking her air-tank regulator in the process. As she later described it, "all of Lake Michigan poured down my throat and I breathed water."

Five minutes later, her diving companions reached her and hauled her to the surface, beginning mouth-to-mouth resuscitation. Two minutes later, she went into cardiac arrest. The Coast Guard rushed to the scene with a pressurized aircraft as soon as they were notified about the accident and the young diver was flown to a University of Michigan clinic where she was diagnosed as having every diving problem imaginable: cold water near-drowning, decompression sickness, suspected air embolism and post-cardiopulmonary arrest. Within hours after the attending physician started his treatment, the diver was alert and doing well; after a few days of observation, she returned to her graduate studies.

Most physicians who work with cold water near-drowning victims believe that resuscitation and survival are made possible by a number of factors. Among the events which occur are a very rapid cooling of the brain, a sudden slowing of all body processes and a drastic reduction in oxygen requirements. These actions usually occur at a time when there is an adequate supply of oxygen in the blood. Because of the sharp drop in oxygen demand, the body is able to survive for a limited time on the "reserve" left in the blood.

The dive reflex is but one of many responses the body has to protect itself from the effects of cooling. As we explore hypothermia, we will find that the body combats the cold in some very complex and intriguing ways. We are confident that understanding these biological processes will help the reader avoid being like the man described in Jack London's hypothermia "classic:"

He was quick and alert in the things of life, but only in the things, and not in the significance. Fifty degrees below zero meant eighty-odd degrees of frost. Such frost impressed him as being cold and uncomfortable, and that was all. It did not lead him to meditate upon his fraility as a creature of temperature, and upon man's fraility in general, able to live within certain narrow limits of heat and cold; and from there on it did not lead him to the conjectural field of immortality and man's place in the universe. Fifty degrees below zero stood for a bite of frost that hurt and that must be guarded against by the use of mittens, ear flaps, warm moccasins and thick socks. Fifty degrees below zero was to him precisely fifty degrees below zero. That there should be anything more to it than that was a thought that never entered his head.

TO BUILD A FIRE
Jack London

CHAPTER 2

Hypothermia and Thermoregulation

Humans can go without water for days at a time and do without food for several weeks, if need be, but they cannot do without warmth for more than a few hours.

Some heat, not too much, not too little, is absolutely necessary for survival. If the body's temperature balance is upset for even a few hours, the odds for survival diminish greatly. Although we may think of our day-to-day need for warmth chiefly as a matter of comfort, heat is really the prime force that keeps each and every cell alive and functioning.

While cold is a universal concern, most people know very little about the role body temperature plays in health and survival. Few are aware of the many ways to protect themselves against the danger of cold and are familiar with the appropriate procedures to follow should they or someone else suffer life-threatening exposure to the cold.

One reason the ordinary citizen knows so little about the cold is that only recently have scientists themselves shown much interest in human thermoregulation in the cold. *Thermoregulation* is the process(es) by which the body regulates and maintains its own temperature within a 1.8–3.6°F (1–2°C) range. While survival in severely cold temperatures has always been a challenge to mankind, and while inquiring minds have long sought to master or at least to adapt to the environment, systematic studies of bodily

9

response to cold temperatures did not occur until the late 1930s.

Regrettable though it is, it was not until some of Hitler's military doctors conducted their "experiments" in the concentration camps at Dachau that data were compiled on human endurance at low temperatures. So disgusted were most scientists by Hitler's undertakings, that the data were treated as "untouchable" for many years. Only much later did technical references to it creep into the medical literature. Even then, researchers apologized for using the data, explaining that they had done so only because no other sources of information existed.

The Korean War, the conflict in Afghanistan, the United States and Soviet space programs, oil exploration in the North Sea, off the coast of Alaska and in America, and the explosion of interest in outdoor sports have all prompted scientists and physicians to initiate new research into thermoregulation in the cold. Today, several universities and major medical centers, as well as various military agencies, have research programs under way.

One major fact all this research has shown is that thermoregulation in the cold involves many different body systems, such as the circulatory system, the respiratory system, the nervous system and others. These systems work together in a coordinated fashion to keep the body as close as possible to its "optimal" temperature of 98.6°F (37°C).

The term *optimal* is used because virtually every cell in the body functions most efficiently at 98.6°F (37°C). Heat is produced within the body by each of the many thousands of individual cells. Some of that heat energy is retained by the body; the rest is discharged in a variety of ways. If the body gets excessively warm or excessively cold, body functions are impaired, cells are damaged and eventually the life process is halted.

Thus, while the body can easily accommodate slight variations (up or down 1.8–3.6°F or 1–2°C) for short periods of time, should body temperature vary significantly above or below that optimal level for very long, health and well-being are endangered.

Since heat is both required and produced at the cellular level, and since the environment variously acts as both a warming and a cooling force, the body must be able to regulate the distribution of heat throughout the head and neck, the trunk and the limbs. Depending on individual needs at any given time, the body must be able to generate heat, retain heat and discharge heat; these processes must be balanced and coordinated in such a way that the cells can be maintained at their optimal thermal level. The body has numerous mechanisms that are in coordination to counteract either extreme cold or excessive heat.

It is this process of coordination that is called *thermoregulation* and, as has been noted, everything functions normally so long as the thermoregulatory process is able to remain centered on 98.6°F (37°C). When body temperatures rise or fall significantly above or below that level, the disruption of bodily processes can very quickly become a severe threat to survival.

One particularly interesting feature of thermoregulation is the fact that the central body, or *core,* temperature (brain, spinal cord, heart, lungs and thorax) and the *peripheral* temperature (limbs and skin) are both "set" at approximately 98.6°F (37°C). However, while peripheral, and especially skin, temperature can vary greatly without serious consequences, even a 2 or 3°F change in core temperature can have severe consequences. Helping to protect the body's core are two outer layers, the skeletal and the skin.

As mentioned, scientists and physicians use the term *hypothermia* to refer to the subnormal temperature of the body and its physiological condition caused when it is unable to maintain an adequate level of warmth for normal body function. Hypothermia can occur in a variety of circumstances and can be caused by interaction of numerous factors, among them cold air, cold water, old age, inadequate nutrition, alcohol, injury and a host of others. A physically fit skin diver working at 40 feet below the surface, a child falling into a mountain lake, a deer hunter having a frequent "nip" on his stand and an elderly woman in her home are *all* potential victims of hypothermia Whatever the

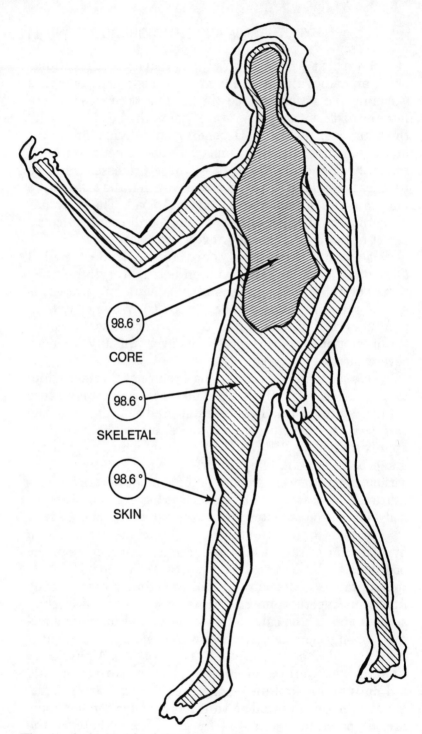

The body in its ideal thermal state.

circumstances and whatever the intervening factors, the essential danger occurs as the body loses its thermoregulatory ability to keep its temperature centered on 98.6°F. Unless that temperature is restored in an orderly, systematic fashion, individual body systems will fail progressively until the victim dies.

Physicians find themselves faced with victims of two types of hypothermia which are life-threatening:

Primary accidental hypothermia is defined as a significant decrease [usually greater than 3.6°F (2°C)] in *central body or core temperature.* This decrease is virtually always caused by exposure to the cold or to chilling conditions. In order for the body to muster all of its resources in combating this cold threat, it is assumed that the victim must be in normal health and that his or her body is functioning properly. Primary accidental hypothermia can arise from cold water immersion, exposure to cold air, whether it be dry or humid, deep water diving and a variety of other circumstances.

Secondary accidental hypothermia is also defined as a significant decrease [usually greater than 3.6°F (2°C)] in body-core temperature, but in this case one or more of the processes which the body uses to maintain its temperature is malfunctioning.

Typically, this type of condition arises when there has been some alteration of either the nervous or the cardiovascular systems. However, as noted in Chapter 5, there is an enormous number of diseases, drugs, debilitating conditions and other disorders which *predispose,* or make, the victim *more susceptible* to hypothermia. For example, strokes or degenerative diseases of the nervous system will alter the body's ability to maintain warmth. Other types of health problems also can affect its ability to direct blood flow from one area of the body to another.

While the effects on the body are often similar, the chief difference between these two types is that in the case of primary accidental hypothermia, the impact of the cold on the body is "causing" the problem or creating the threat to life. In the case of secondary accidental hypothermia, there is some other factor at work which *predisposes* the victim to hypothermia. Clearly, there are many factors which can contribute to excessive chilling and which can prevent a person from maintaining the body heat he needs for survival. In prolonged and severe situations, hypothermia can produce effects ranging from shivering to cardiac arrhythmias and death. However, in most cases, preventive measures or proper clinical treatment can sharply reduce the risks.

We might also acknowledge that there are several other types of hypothermia.

1. *Artificial* or *clinical hypothermia* involves the *controlled* cooling of the body for purposes of medical treatment or research.

2. *Hibernation* is a torpid condition in which certain animals pass the winter months. True hibernators, such as woodchucks and ground squirrels, allow their body temperature to drop near the freezing point. They have very low metabolism, respiration, and heart rates. Partial hibernators, such as bears and skunks, undergo reduced physiological activity, but they are not comatose.

3. *Estivation* is comparable to hibernation, except that it is found in desert animals, such as the Mohave ground squirrel, and it involves a quiescent, torpid state during the summer months.

In order to understand and prevent the occurrence of accidental hypothermia, and to treat hypothermia victims, it is necessary to be familiar with the ways the body has of regulating its temperature; that is, we must understand the process of thermoregulation.

Thermoregulation is controlled by the brain, the spinal cord and the extensive network of nerves which runs throughout the body. The brain is a highly sophisticated, computer-like control center which directs two separate systems. The first of these is the voluntary or somatic nervous system. As its name suggests, this system enables us to act according to our own volition or will, and with it we evaluate a situation and consciously decide, for example, whether to put on a hat, build a fire or move to the tropics in order to stay warm.

The second system is the involuntary or autonomic nervous system. This system controls all internal organs and blood vessels in the body. It also controls the secretion of adrenalin from the adrenal medulla and it *automatically* responds in very specific ways when confronted with certain situations. The part of the brain called the *hypothalamus* directs most of the responses of the autonomic nervous system, whereas the *cerebral cortex* directs most of our voluntary actions. If we fall into icy water, the heart races and the blood pressure increases. (We don't stop to think about these actions, they just happen. Unless we have mastered some discipline, such as yoga, we seldom have any control over these autonomic responses.)

The nervous system controls the thermal generating and regulatory mechanisms of the body, and, as said, its temperature varies considerably [1.8°F (1°C) or more] during a 24-hour period. This rhythmical change is physiologic. As we get older the body temperature fluctuations may no longer be synchronized with activity so that instead of being cooler when we are asleep, we may be cooler during the waking hours.

Thermoregulation would not be possible were it not for the fact that the nervous system enables the brain to monitor virtually every function in the body, one of which is temperature. The nervous system is easily able to detect even minute variations from the optimal temperature of 98.6°F (37°C). Whenever deviations from that temperature are sensed, both the autonomic and the voluntary nervous systems are brought into action. Typically, we respond with conscious actions, such as putting on a coat, but at an unconscious level the brain calls many other bodily systems (respiratory, circulatory, endocrine, etc.) into play in a highly coordinated effort to protect our lives.

(As an aside, it should be emphasized that it is absolutely essential that all rescue and clinical interventions, as well as preventive measures, be designed to compliment and work in harmony with the thermoregulatory process—to do otherwise may accentuate the danger rather than reduce it. The reasons behind this cautionary note will become apparent in a later chapter.)

Our thermoregulatory processes, controlled by the nervous system are committed to maintaining the optimal 98.6°F temperature, above or below which the various systems work together to generate and conserve heat or to discharge it. Thus, to adjust to too much heat or too little, the nervous system continually monitors both the brain/heart temperature and the skin/muscle temperature and compares the two. It is this comparison which dictates the way the body will respond to cold or heat stress.

For example, if the skin is chilled rapidly (as occurs when we jump into a cool lake), that information is relayed immediately to the brain and spinal cord. The dropping skin temperature is compared with the temperature of the heart and brain, and the nervous system activates various processes which will generate and conserve heat. In this example, the most notable response is *behavioral*; we would probably spontaneously jump up and down in shallow water or start swimming furiously to "get used to the water." Conversely, if the brain senses that the skin temperature is increasing, it will activate certain processes which will cause the body to discharge heat. Thus, as we lie in the sun, our skin gets warm and we begin to sweat—a cooling process. While there are many other, far more complicated ways the body regulates its temperature, shivering, exercising, sweating and even moving into the shade are basic examples of thermoregulation. Our front-line defense, then, is usually a behavioral reaction, in which the initial response to temperature stress is to alter our environment, either by taking some direct protective action or by moving away from the source of stress.

So, when we get too warm we may turn on an air conditioner or a fan, move to a shady spot or drink a cool beverage. When we feel ourselves getting too cold, we may slip on additional clothing, move to a warmer location or snuggle up to someone else. It's only common sense, you might say. Perhaps, but actually the brain has initiated this behavior after having determined the presence of some form of thermal stress. This determination was made via thousands of thermal receptors; specialized parts of the nervous system located at strategic points throughout the body, including the skin, internal organs, the spinal cord and certain areas of the brain. Even the tongue and the respiratory system have their share of thermal receptors. There are separate sensors for heat and for cold, and when either type is activated by a temperature stimulus these specialized nerve endings begin to send electrical signals to the brain. Just how or where that thermal information is processed in the brain is not completely understood, but scientists do know that the resulting electrical and/or neurochemical messages are transmitted immediately, thus initiating an appropriate response, be it shivering, sweating, or a change in the rate of blood flow.

To better understand these receptors, consider the analogy of a house. For each person there is a temperature at which he or she is most comfortable. To keep your house at that desired temperature, you can use a furnace and air conditioning unit with a blower or "pumping" mechanism and a thermostat. The thermostat is a thermal receptor—it senses temperature and, with its electrical switching capability, turns the heating or cooling unit on or off.

Many older homes have a single thermostat and, as a consequence, room temperature may differ throughout the house. In the summer, the upper level rooms on the south side will be warmer than the ground level rooms on the north side, and the basement will be yet another temperature.

Many modern homes are built more like the human body. They have thermostats throughout, and individual rooms or sections can be heated or cooled independently. Some also have a computer which senses and maintains the desired temperature of every room. This temperature is called the set point.

The thermal sensing system of the human body is

infinitely more complex than that of a house, but the principle is the same. All of our bodily "rooms" are constantly monitored and warmed or cooled, depending on our needs. Most of the time we are unconscious of this thermal sensing operation, but much of the "information" can be called into consciousness on a split-second's notice. For example, although you probably weren't thinking until this moment about whether the big toe on your right foot is warm or cold, on demand your brain would bring that information into your awareness immediately.

Although the body uses the brain and its thermal sensors in much the same way that we use thermostats and a minicomputer in a modern house, neither the brain nor the thermal sensors have the capability of producing or transmitting heat. In the next chapter we will see that heat is continually produced in the body as a result of chemical processes at the level of individual cells. Those chemical activities are referred to as metabolic reactions. The metabolic rate indicates the extent to which heat is being produced in the body. In the house analogy, the furnace is the component which heats the water that is then pumped to the radiators.

Some heat "moves" through the body simply because cells are in contact with each other, but the chief mechanism for heat distributing is the circulatory system, of which the heart can be compared with the pump or blower in a home heating system.

Just as the pump in a hot water home heating system moves hot water through a network of pipes, the heart moves warm blood through a network of arteries, veins, capillaries and superficial blood vessels, and although the heart is constantly working, if its pumping ability is decreased, its ability to keep the body warm will also decrease.

The major difference between these two distribution systems is that the body uses a much more complicated and efficient network of "pipes." Because we have what might be considered "circulatory sensors," similar to our thermal sensors, the brain is able to monitor heart rate, blood flow to the brain, blood flow to the extremities, blood pressure, and so on. In fact, the autonomic nervous system includes nerves which wrap around most major blood vessels for the specific purpose of channeling or directing blood flow from one part of the body to another. This process of directing blood flow is called *shunting,* and the nerves which control it are so powerful that they can virtually stop all blood flow to a hand, arm or leg, for example. The *cardiovascular* (the pumping system) plays a critical role in thermoregulation because the blood it moves serves as the major agent for heat transfer within the body. If an area is too hot, the blood serving it is transferred to a "cooler" place, usually the skin, as the autonomic nervous system opens up superficial blood vessels.

An unsung hero in this process is the body's vast array of blood vessels and its unique ability to change their diameter. Operating at the command of the autonomic nervous system and the direct control of the hormone epinephrine, arteries are able to expand or constrict their diameters depending on the need for more or less heat in various body parts. This action of constriction enables the body to shunt blood from one region to another and is the cornerstone of thermoregulation. If the body core temperature is too high, the arteries serving the skin and extremities will dilate, or open, to allow the warm blood to move near the surface of the skin where excessive heat can be dissipated; this process of expansion is called *vasodilatation.* If, on the other hand, core body heat must be conserved, the autonomic nervous system diverts blood flow from the skin by closing off the superficial blood vessels; this process which operates on internal blood vessels as well, is called vasoconstriction. So effective are these processes that if the need arises, blood flow to the finger, for example, can be reduced 99% by vasoconstriction.

Vasodilatation, vasoconstriction, and shunting will reappear again and again in our examination of hypothermia. It is because of these mechanisms, along with the network of thermal sensors, that the brain is able to regulate temperature throughout the body so quickly and accurately.

To demonstrate these processes for yourself, place the tip of one index finger into a glass of ice water for 30–60 seconds and then remove it. Place the tip of that finger and the tip of the second finger on your cheek about 1–1.5 inches apart. One finger will feel cold, the other warm. Move the fingers away from your cheek for approximately 60 seconds and then replace them. They will both feel "normal." In that short time, the autonomic nervous system has activated several procedures, chief among them vasodilatation, by selectively rewarming just that fingertip without increasing heat production or distribution anywhere else in the finger or hand.

The brain thus regulates the temperature of the body in much the same way you would heat a cold house if you were faced with a limited fuel supply. When winter is with us, we must do what we can to conserve fuel. One of the first conservation measures would be to shut off the heat to various parts of the house. Rooms which have marginal utilitarian value are simple closed off. Those of greatest use and importance, such as the kitchen, are the last to be shut off.

The brain acts in much the same way when it is subjected to cold stress. The colder the environment becomes, or the longer we are exposed to even moderate cooling conditions, the harder the body must work to keep itself centered on 98.6°F (37°C). As the body works harder to maintain its thermal balance, physiological stress is increased. As this stress increases, the body's energy resources are depleted at an even greater rate. With its furnaces going "full blast," the body runs the risk of completely exhausting its energy reserves.

To avoid these threats to survival, the brain establishes priorities and diverts energy from those structures of least importance. The brain and heart are given highest priority; other internal organs are next, followed by the limbs and outer extremities. As the core temperature drops, the brain struggles to maintain all parts in good working order, but when the chips are down, it is fully capable of making seemingly ruthless, sacrificial decisions; to do otherwise would hasten death. Thus the brain stops blood flow to the expendable extremities first in order to maintain vital core temperature. If in the process of prolonged vasoconstriction a foot is lost, but core temperature, and hence life, is maintained, then the price is small in comparison.

Of course, there is much more to thermoregulation than having the brain choose to sacrifice a foot. The nervous system first senses the endangering cold and begins telegraphing that message to the center of consciousness. Once we are conscious of the cold, we take actions to keep warm. We put on extra clothing if it is available; we move around briskly, stamp our feet and clap our hands; we build fires and shelters; we curl into a ball, thereby reducing the amount of body surface exposed. Depending on the circumstances, there are many ways we can consciously react to the threat of cold.

But conscious behavioral reactions aren't always sufficient. Therefore, as insurance, while the brain is notifying the voluntary nervous system of cold stress, the autonomic nervous system is also reacting. Nerves which control the heart will cause it to increase its rate, and blood vessels will be instructed to direct warm blood away from the cold area. Respiration will also be increased. As extra insurance, the cold stress will also trigger the endocrine system, a complex group of specialized cells and glands in the body that secretes chemical messengers into the blood like a counterpart to our "electrical" nervous system. The hormone epnephrine (adrenaline), for example, causes the heart to increase the rate of its pumping action.

In addition, if the conscious response to temperature stress involves physical activity, the generation of heat and energy by the cells, will be increased as the body converts glycogen stored in the tissues into glucose, the form of energy used by the cells for fuel. This reaction occurs slowly and is of benefit in acute cold stress. One result, for example, is that the muscles will begin shivering, a tremor-like movement which in itself generates heat.

While the nervous system is engaged in juggling all of these defensive and protective measures, it must sort out an immense quantity of information and keep all of the systems in balance. Respiration, ventilation, and circulation must be synchronized; the endocrine system, the neuromuscular system and even the digestive system must each be placed "on alert" and pitched into action when necessary. As these systems are all brought into play in response to the cold, the body undergoes a double stress: the first, obviously, is from the cold itself. The second is from the strain of defense. Each defensive action taken further stresses the body and can be continued for only a limited period. For example, shivering usually ceases once the body's core temperature reaches 86°F (30°C), and is an effective heat generating activity only until the energy stores are depleted.

The effects of hypothermia occur initially as a result of an "overload" on our biological defense mechanisms. Frostbite can have an early, localized impact that can be quite serious, but it is not life threatening in and of itself. Only much later, when all systems have failed or "closed down," does hypothermia's ultimate impact, death from exposure or freezing, occur.

However, an extremely important point to keep in mind is this: as the body moves through the various levels of hypothermia, nearly all of its systems are progressively slowed down, many of them to the point where the victim *appears* completely lifeless. This can be very deceiving. Remarkably, the severe chilling can have a beneficial effect *if* the victim is rewarmed early enough and in the appropriate manner. There are cases on record where persons who were "frozen to death" were discovered and subsequently brought back to normal health.

The key to such astonishing rescue efforts is the courage, wisdom and skill of the rescue workers who first found the victims and the clinicians who treated them. Furthermore, the rewarming and revival efforts were undertaken in a way that complimented those steps the body had already taken to protect itself. Had the victims been rewarmed too rapidly, had fluids been administered too early, the victims might have died from cardiac failure or from insulin shock. Many other complications can also occur in rewarming, thus the need for a comprehensive understanding of the body's *total* response to cold when dealing with situations which are potentially hypothermic.

CHAPTER 3

The Biology of Body Heat

One of the most common precautions one can take to prevent hypothermia is to be well-fed before entering a cold environment. The reasoning behind this statement is the fact that it is from food that we obtain the fuel our body uses to produce heat. In a word, food intake = heat loss + work output + energy storage.

If we consume enough food to handle the heat loss and work (energy) output requirements, then the remaining food energy is stored in the body. Obviously, however, if our food intake does not match the heat loss and work output, then the body must draw on its stored energy reserves. This latter process is time consuming and it is not an effective way to produce heat for one's immediate needs.

The first section of this chapter will deal with the processes involved in transforming food (carbohydrates, proteins and fats) into the energy we need to stay alive.

Previously we learned that heat is essential for life and that the body has some fairly complex mechanisms which it uses to sense and regulate its internal and external temperatures. When the brain senses that the body is too warm, it is able to implement such cooling processes as sweating, vasodilatation and having a cold drink. If the body is becoming too cold, the brain engages various heat production and heat conservation mechanisms such as shivering, vasoconstriction or moving closer to the fire. Since hypothermia is fundamentally a thermal, or temperature, stress on the body, we must examine the ways that the body produces, conserves and discharges heat if we are to understand the problems of subnormal body temperatures.

An exploration of the biology of body heat must begin at the level of the individual cell. The body is comprised of literally thousands of cells and hundreds of different cell types. There are different types of cells for bone, muscle tissue, nerves, organs and for each of the many other components of the body. Regardless of its type, each cell must "look after itself" with respect to obtaining nutrients, oxygen, water, and various other cellular compounds. The circulatory system is solely responsible for delivering these required substances to the cells, but the cells themselves must take what they need from the blood in order to synthesize proteins (used to rebuild and maintain their cellular structure) and to "extract" energy.

Energy enters into the picture because *cells are able to function only as a result of chemical reactions* and energy is both a necessary ingredient for and a by-product of every chemical reaction that occurs. For this reason many scientists refer to the body as an incredibly complex chemical factory; ultimately, everything we think and do is a result of a chemical reaction which has occured somewhere in the body.

In a sense, we are driven by our cells. Each individual cell is like a tiny machine which runs compulsively. To function properly, the cell needs glucose, water, oxygen and a variety of other chemical substances. But, since each cell cannot directly obtain those compounds from the external environment, the body has developed a variety of specialized support systems, with specialized cells, each of which performs certain tasks which are coordinated with the functions of other systems. Thus, the muscular system enables us to find and obtain food; the digestive system "processes" it; the circulatory system delivers it and our liver and kidneys de-toxify unusable by-products. All of these functions are coordinated by the brain and the nervous system, as well as by the endocrine system. The life process involves many other systems in addition to those mentioned.

Carrying out these life processes, in addition to their own internal "housekeeping" functions, requires that our cells remain in a constant state of activity. Such activity may increase or decrease at various times, but no cell is ever truly inactive unless it has died.

The word *activity* has been used rather loosely thus far. What it really refers to is chemical activity and the term *metabolism* is used specifically to refer to the body's total set of chemical reactions.

Interestingly, the term metabolism comes from a Greek word meaning to *change*. Thus, *metabolism* draws attention to the fact that the body changes raw components into the energy needed for life processes and into the material needed to repair and replace cells. That raw material comes from food. The conversion of food into energy and cellular material is the cornerstone of heat production in the human body.

There are many different kinds of food, but all foods are composed of one or more of three building blocks: proteins, carbohydrates, and lipids (or fats). Food is further classified according to its energy value. Fatty foods have more energy per gram of food than carbohydrates, for example. The amount of energy available in food is rated using a measurement called calories.

A Calorie (note the capital "C") is the amount of heat necessary to increase 1 liter (about one quart) of water one degree Centigrade. On the other hand, 1 calorie (note the lower case "c") is the amount of heat needed to raise 1 milliliter of water 1 degree Centigrade. A thousand small calories are equal to 1 Calorie. Scientists call this big Calorie a kilocalorie.

When diet books refer to counting calories, they are referring to kilocalories. Thus, a four-inch slice of blueberry pie contains 350 kilocalories (or Calories) and is therefore capable of producing enough heat to raise the temperature of 88 gallons of water 1 degree Centigrade. Calorie determination is made using a device known as a "bomb" calorimeter. In essence a measured amount of the foodstuff is placed in a well-insulated box and "exploded," hence the name "bomb." The amount of heat produced by this instantaneous combustion of the food is then measured using a water bath and a very precise thermometer. Having that information, we can say, for example, that the small pat of butter you put on your toast every morning has enough energy stored in it to melt 2 pounds of ice and bring it to a boil.

Talking about a pat of butter having that much energy in it makes us pause for a moment to consider just what we mean when we talk about energy. Within that small pat of butter is an enormous amount of chemical energy. Fats are highly complex chemical structures which have thousands of atoms bound together as molecules and hundreds of molecules bound together as, say, a pat of butter. Thus, when those fatty molecules are broken down by the chemical actions of digestion, chemical energy is released.

The three basic food types differ in the amount of energy they have available for release. One gram of carbohydrates yields 5.10 Calories, one gram of protein, 5.6 Calories and one gram of pure fat, 9.45 Calories. (Because our bodies cannot break down food completely, at least not as efficiently as the "bomb" calorimeter does, our ingested carbohydrates and proteins have a usable Caloric value of 5.0, while fats have a value of 9.0.) Obviously, fats (or lipids) have the highest amount of energy.

It is worth noting that the fruit–nut–chocolate type of trail mixes carried by many backpackers, hikers and mountain climbers contains some of all three types of food groups. These rations thus provide both short- and long- term energy needs.

In our modern, highly technological, society we typically shun food high in Calories, but in situations of stress, high-Caloric foods are valued because that energy is available to the body as it reacts to protect itself. Since stress is, by definition, something that is *ultimately* life threatening, any food which provides us with the energy we might need to fight or escape is valuable.

This point is important with reference to hypothermia, because it is one of those life-threatening stresses. Vast quantities of energy are required to combat heat loss, and individuals who consistently eat foods having low-Caloric values will be less capable of resisting the stress of hypothermia.

So what happens to that food we eat?

Depending on a variety of factors, such as our personal physiological make-up, our health status, our level of exertion, etc., our ingested food will be metabolized slowly or, if need be, more rapidly.

As was noted earlier, all of us have a minimal level of activity, some metabolic rate at which our particular body operates. Scientists refer to this as our basal metabolic rate. This basal metabolic rate (BMR) is usually measured in people by determining precisely the amount of oxygen consumed by a person who has not eaten for twelve hours. The person lies quietly for a while, relaxing to bring the muscles and mind to a resting status and then oxygen consumption is measured. Why measure oxygen when we are interested in basal metabolism? Because it is well established that when one liter of oxygen is consumed in the combustion of protein, carbohydrates, and lipids, approximately five Calories are produced. Knowing how many liters of oxygen a person is consuming thus enables scientists to determine how many Calories are being used.

When we talk about Calories being used, what we are really saying is that chemical energy is being released in the body. Some of that energy continues to exist as chemical energy, other energy is transformed into heat. The transfer and transformation of energy starts in the digestive system and (for our purpose) ends up at the individual cellular level.

Within our bodies, most injested carbohydrates are converted into glucose. It is this glucose which is used primarily by the cells for energy. If the cells do not use the glucose, it is stored as glycogen in the muscle and the liver. Since glucose is the preferred fuel source directly available to the cells, a constant supply of glucose in the blood is essential for optimal functioning; the brain, especially, must have a constant supply of this important commodity. *Without glucose (as well as oxygen and heat) all bodily func-*

tions cease. When the amount of glucose in the bloodstream drops to a certain level, the body begins to regenerate blood glucose supply from liver glycogen stores.

When fats are digested, fatty acids and glycerol are produced. These are then recombined to form triglycerides (a type of lipid), which are subsequently stored in the muscles and fatty tissues. When needed, the triglycerides are broken down into "free fatty acids," which can then be converted into energy by the cells.

Most people know that glucose and fats are important as fuels for the body, but few are aware that these compounds are only important precursors of the real workhorse, ATP (adenosine triphosphate). ATP is the end product of the metabolism of food. It is from the high-energy chemical bonds in ATP that cells actually "get" the energy which enables them to function. To describe just how ATP transfers this chemical energy is beyond the scope of this book. The release of energy stored in ATP results in what we recognize as movement, thought, secretion or any of the other functions performed by our cells. To read this page requires that the eyeballs scan back and forth across the page. The direct energy enabling the muscle cells to move the eyeballs is provided by ATP. Likewise, when cross-country skiing or riding a bicycle, ATP is used to contract and relax your muscles.

Cells burn carbohydrates and fat in the presence of oxygen to form ATP. The oxygen is delivered by the circulatory system which, in turn, has obtained oxygen from the respiratory system. Suppose then, that you stopped breathing: could you still use the glucose in your blood to keep the cells functioning? Yes! For a limited period of time the cells can utilize glucose (but not fatty acids) to synthesize ATP when oxygen is absent. This capability is limited, however, and the amount of ATP produced is only 10% of what it would be were oxygen present. Certain cells are able to synthesize ATP without oxygen much more efficiently than others. Muscle cells, for example, can continue to produce ATP without oxygen longer than brain cells.

How does all of this relate to heat production?

In daily life we take in a certain amount of energy in the form of food. Foodstuffs are, after all, nothing more than various compounds whose molecules contain stored chemical energy. Those molecules are broken down by the digestive system and synthesized into new molecules in the body. The processes which break down and synthesize chemical compounds are simple chemical reactions. At the basis of all these chemical reactions is our utilization of glucose, fatty acids, and oxygen in the formation of ATP. As we regenerate ATP, we also produce heat. Since there are literally thousands of minute reactions occurring every second, there is a tremendous amount of heat being produced in the body. In fact, there is so much heat being produced by the body that we might easily, and not inappropriately, refer to it as a metabolic furnace.

We seldom stop to realize just how dependent we are on the heat generated by our bodies. A vivid illustration of the relationship between heat and food is provided by the hunger strikers in Northern Ireland. Noting that by the third day of starvation most strikers were already consuming energy stored as fat, a scientist observed that the protesters were suffering from lowered body temperatures and that they spent virtually all of their time in bed under several layers of sheepskin rugs. Although the environmental conditions in the prison were relatively warm and protective, the strikers were still suffering from hypothermia. Ultimately, the body literally digests itself and death by starvation results from a complete breakdown of multiple body systems.

Before leaving the topic of metabolism, we might take note of one other interesting aspect of food which is related to heat production. Most people have noticed that they feel warmer after having eaten a meal. Such observations are most frequent after people have eaten large quantities of protein. Scientists generally attribute this after-dinner warmth to the fact that certain amino acids (the basic compounds in proteins) are not easily metabolized. As a consequence, many individual chemical reactions take place following ingestion of such substances. With all of those reactions taking place, it is only to be expected that an excessive amount of heat will also be produced. This process is referred to as the *Specific Dynamic Action* of foods. Carbohydrates and lipids produce some heat in this way, but protein has the highest Specific Dynamic Action.

In reference to this last point, it should be noted that these metabolic actions also *require* a considerable amount of energy. Thus, a hypothermic individual might not have expendable energy reserves to "waste" on digesting protein to create body heat. Glucose, except in certain situations, is much more likely to be effectively used by the hypothermic victim.

Additional heat, sometimes in great amounts, is produced once we begin to do work. Walking, reading, writing, chopping wood, and stamping our feet are examples of "work." All such activities, since they involve the transformation of chemical energy into mechanical energy (such as chopping wood), produce some increase in our metabolic rate. In the process, heat is generated.

Thus, while stamping our feet when we are cold may not serve to advance the cause of civilization, the warmth it creates does serve the needs of the organism. When we are cold, clapping our hands, building a shelter and swimming to shore are examples of "work" which has survival value—through the heat produced, if nothing else.

To summarize heat production, then, our basal metabolism and the metabolic activity resulting from "work" are the dominant methods by which heat is produced in the body. Our metabolic furnace can produce tremendous quantities of heat, some of which is used to maintain the cells in their optimal thermal environment of 98.6°F (37°C). The rest of that heat must be dissipated because the body can only store a limited amount of heat. We generally refer to this dissipation as heat loss.

In most situations, some heat loss is to be expected and, indeed, is essential. However, in cold situations where heat loss is accelerated (i.e., when more heat is being lost than the body is able to replace), the loss becomes a threat to life.

Surprisingly, there are only four ways the body can lose heat; an examination of these physical factors in heat loss is the next step in understanding hypothermia.

In the previous section we examined the production of heat by cells, a process which is technically called *cellular thermogenesis*. We say that the body is much like a furnace: the "pilot light" is constantly burning and a minimal amount of heat is being produced continually. Physiologists and physicians refer to this as the basal metabolic rate. As our muscles, organs and glands function, they require additional energy and in response, our metabolic furnace fires itself up.

The human body acts like a sleeve around that furnace. The heat resulting from metabolic activity is produced within that sleeve. Although some 30% of that heat is used to maintain the organs, glands and nervous system at their optimal temperature of 98.6°F (37°C), some means must exist for the body to discharge the remaining 70%. If the "heat sleeve" could not vent itself, the system would literally burn up.

In this section, then, we will review the mechanisms by which the body discharges its excess heat. Understanding the mechanisms for heat exchange (and, therefore, heat loss) is of critical importance when looking at hypothermia since virtually all hypothermic conditions represent situations in which heat loss is accelerated.

Heat is much like electricity; everyone has an intuitive sense of what it is, but few people can really explain it. Technically, heat is a characteristic of electromagnetic waves; these waves are a phenomenon resulting from the movement of electrons in atoms. Since all atoms have electrons in motion, all atoms generate some amount of heat. Theoretically, there is a state, called absolute zero (−273°C), in which all electron activity is halted, but that state has never been created in the laboratory. In the cold depths of outer space, the temperature is approximately three degrees above absolute zero.

Like electricity, heat behaves according to certain laws.

One such law is that when electrons are excited, they move faster, thus creating more heat. Electrons can be excited by chemical reactions, friction and many other ways.

Another law or property of heat is that it always flows along a gradient. That's a complicated way of saying that heat, like water, "seeks its own level." Whenever a warm entity is surrounded or is in contact with any substance which is cooler than it is, heat will move from the warm object toward its cooler counterpart. If you place your warm hand on an ice cube, what you feel is heat rushing from your hand to the ice cube.

RADIATION

Radiation is a process whereby electromagnetic energy (including heat) is able to travel through space at the speed of light. Light is, in fact, a form of electromagnetic energy that is visible. Infrared, ultraviolet and radio waves are the same type of energy, but they are not visible without special lenses or other sensing equipment; neither are the waves generated by a microwave oven, but they can certainly transmit heat to another object.

As we noted, all objects have electromagnetic energy and so they all radiate energy. At high temperatures, a common light bulb emits a visible light and infrared radiation. At low temperatures (when it's "turned off"), it radiates primarily infrared energy.

The human body both emits and receives various forms of radiant energy. At this moment your body is radiating infrared heat to the walls around you if they are colder than you are. Because of the principle that heat moves along a gradient, the waves *from* the warmer object dominate. Thus, if a person with a skin temperature of 80.6°F (27°C) was standing nude in a room which had an air temperature of 72°F (22°C), he would lose a lot of heat as a result of his radiated infrared waves. The amount of heat loss due to radiation depends on surface area and the difference between skin and air temperatures (the thermal gradient). Radiation is an important consideration with respect to cold temperatures since we lose body heat via radiation from the body surface, while we also gain heat by the same process, as from reflected radiation from the snow, heat from fires, etc.

Some enterprising individuals have attempted to minimize heat loss by radiation by placing a layer of aluminum foil inside their winter garments. Aluminum foil is a powerful reflector of infrared radiation. Most backpackers who have tried this method of heat conservation have discovered that they sweated too much because the aluminum foil would not allow for evaporation. Although the idea of repelling infrared radiation is a good attempt at minimizing heat loss, it actually increases the chances for hypothermia because it minimizes evaporation and leaves the person very wet.

It is important to keep in mind the fact that *everything* radiates heat, but if you are cold, you will benefit only if you are in the vicinity of objects which are radiating more heat than you are. With respect to your own body, heat is radiated from finger to finger and from leg to leg. If you are cold and you assume the fetal position, some of your radiating surface areas will be radiating to each other and you will be minimizing heat loss.

CONDUCTION

Heat transfer via this process *requires actual physical contact between two objects*. The transfer of heat in this way thus involves the interaction of molecules and atoms. Radiant heat can move through a vacuum, but molecules of snow, rock, ice and sand, for example, must be present for conduction to occur.

Conduction also occurs in our bodies. Heat is conducted from our exercising muscles to the skin surface. The heat is further conducted from the skin by a thin layer of air which is present on our skin to objects with which it is in contact. For example, if a person is mildly hypothermic one of the recommended therapies is to take off his wet clothes, dry him off and put him in a sleeping bag with two other persons. The resulting body contact will warm the victim by conduction.

All substances have certain values of thermal conductivity. In other words some objects are better thermal conductors than others. If a substance is a *poor thermal conductor it is a good insulator*. To minimize heat loss you need a good insulator, material that does not conduct heat readily. Values for insulation are expressed in the term of "CLOs." The greater the CLO value, the better the insulation. Feathers and fur have a much higher CLO value than does the typical business suit. Animal fur, for example, has hair that traps air (which is a good insulator) and a hair arrangement which prevents cold air from disturbing the warm air. Another good insulator is human fat. Fat people have built-in insulation. Most women have a thicker subcutaneous fat layer than men and hence have better insulation as well.

On the other hand, good thermal conductors pose special threats. Water has a much higher thermal conductivity than does air. Again, water conducts heat 25 times faster than does air. Although air at 25°F (−4°C) is as cold as water at 25°F (−4°C), the thermal conductivity of water will take heat from the human body much faster than air. Steel conducts even faster than does water and therefore sitting on cold steel such as bleachers, oil rig platforms, ships, etc., is worse than being in cold water, except in cold water a much larger area of the body's surface is exposed to the cold and exposed body surface is an important factor, as we have seen.

CONVECTION

This term refers to a special type of conduction. Conduction *per se* involves only *physical contact* between two or more substances. Convection *is the term used to refer to situations in which one of those substances is in motion*. When air or fluids move over a thermal object, heat is transferred to individual molecules of air (or fluid) which then move out of contact and are replaced by new, cooler molecules which, again, absorb heat by conduction and move out of contact. This circulation process is aided by the propensity of heat to rise; warmed air or fluid is displaced by cooler molecules. We can increase the heat loss due to convection by riding a motorcycle or jogging. Both situations cause wind to stream across the body.

Heat loss via convection depends not only on the thermal difference between the two "objects," but on the physical characteristics of the substances as well. Such factors as viscosity and density will affect the rate at which conduction of heat to the cool substance will occur, as will the speed at which such fluids (or gases) circulate. The surface of the body (or any thermal object) also enters into the process. Fluids and gases move across smooth surfaces more rapidly than over rough surfaces, but rough surfaces create more turbulance. Both speed and turbulance affect the rate at which cooler molecules are brought into contact with the warmer surface.

Convective heat transfer is extremely important. When you are exercising *in a cool environment* your core temperature will begin to rise. This increase in core temperature is transmitted throughout your entire body. As a consequence the blood vessels on the skin are dilated so that the warm blood is cooled by the temperature of the air. Much body heat is lost on a windy day by way of convection. The wind whipping across a person's body will cause heat transfer. Since heat transfer is always from the warmer to the colder object, heat loss is accentuated by convection. This whole concept is described as *wind chill*. There is no question that the wind can chill you. The rate of heat transfer is determined to some extent by the temperature difference, thus the greater the difference between the temperature of a warm jogger and the cold wind the greater the heat loss and the greater the chance for hypothermia.

Cold dry wind has its severe chilling effect because of the rate at which heat and moisture are drawn off. The "wind chill index" is an attempt to quantify the combined effects of air speed, temperature and relative humidity. The colder the wind chill index and the longer one is exposed to it, the greater the likelihood of hypothermia occurring. Because of the efficiency of convection as a heat transfer process, the cold wind becomes a continual heat drain.

The rate at which heat is lost via convection in rapidly

Wind Chill Equivalent Temperature (°F)

Wind Speed (MPH)	Air Temperature (°F)																		
	45	40	35	30	25	20	15	10	5	0	-5	-10	-15	-20	-25	-30	-35	-40	-45
0	69	67	65	62	60	58	55	53	50	48	46	43	41	39	36	34	31	29	27
5	43	37	32	27	22	16	11	6	1	-5	-10	-15	-20	-26	-31	-36	-41	-47	-52
10	34	28	22	16	10	4	-3	-9	-15	-21	-27	-33	-40	-46	-52	-58	-64	-70	-76
15	29	22	16	9	2	-5	-11	-18	-25	-32	-38	-45	-52	-58	-65	-72	-79	-85	-92
20	25	18	11	4	-3	-10	-17	-25	-32	-39	-46	-53	-60	-67	-74	-82	-89	-96	-103
25	23	15	8	0	-7	-15	-22	-29	-37	-44	-52	-59	-66	-74	-81	-89	-96	-104	-111
30	21	13	5	-2	-10	-18	-25	-33	-41	-48	-56	-63	-71	-79	-86	-94	-102	-109	-117
35	19	11	3	-4	-12	-20	-28	-35	-43	-51	-59	-67	-74	-82	-90	-98	-106	-113	-121
40	18	10	2	-6	-14	-22	-29	-37	-45	-53	-61	-69	-77	-85	-93	-101	-108	-116	-124
45	17	9	1	-7	-15	-23	-31	-39	-47	-55	-62	-70	-78	-86	-94	-102	-110	-118	-126

flowing cold water is even higher than it is in cold wind. The reason for this is that water is more dense than air and there are thus more molecules per square centimeter available for contact and heat transfer. For the person who falls into cold water, such recommended safety procedures as hugging the knees or drawing up into a ball represent attempts to reduce the amount of body surface exposed to the chilling waters.

While we have focused on the role of conduction and convection in heat *loss* thus far, the principles of heat loss can be put to good effect when dealing with potentially hypothermic situations. Goosedown outerwear, for example, derives its heat-conserving characteristics from the layer of insulating air created by the three-dimensional structure of the down. (Ordinary feathers are flat and thus fail to create as much air space.) The layer of air is warmed by the body and cooled by the external wind, but like all good insulators, it has a strong buffering effect and little heat is lost from the body.

Wet suits, as used by divers, are also based on the insulating principles afforded by conduction. Wet suits hold a thin layer of water next to the body and the water is warmed by metabolic and shivering heat. The outer surface of the suit resists heat loss through convection to the lake or ocean, while the internal water layer minimizes such heat transfer as does occur. The tighter the fit of the wet suit, the greater its ability to reduce heat loss and to protect against cold water; this is due to the fact that the body has a smaller quantity of water to keep warm and because thin layers of water circulate less than larger quantities. Naturally, if the suit is torn, the internal layer of insulating water is "invaded" by cold water and the suit becomes nothing more than a chilling sleeve. Also, if one compresses any kind of insulator it will lose some of its insulating properties.

Convection and conduction deserve special attention because of the critical heat exchange role they play inside the body. Most people assume that convection and conduction play a large role outside the body, but hardly any inside—such is definitely not the case.

We learned in Chapter 2 that the brain is able to use

vasoconstriction and vasodilatation of arteries to reduce or to increase blood flow to various parts of the body. This shunting process is also used to divert blood flow to, or from, the skin via the superficial blood vessels. In addition, we noted that blood serves as the primary agent for heat transfer within the body; convection is the process which enables blood to serve that crucial role.

In normal circumstances the body's metabolic activity creates thermal energy which originates at the level of individual cells. Some cells (such as those which comprise our intestinal and liver tissue) are more active than others (such as those which make up our fingernails). Likewise, different parts of the body are serviced by a more or less extensive array of blood vessels. In general, areas likely to experience high levels of local metabolic activity are the better served.

Our blood travels through the circulatory system, being distributed through smaller and smaller vessels as it moves to the farthest reaches of the body. Like any other thermal object, blood is subject to the physical laws which govern heat. Thus, when blood moves through the body and comes in contact with tissues which are warmer than the blood itself, heat is transferred to the blood via the process of convection. The blood moves on until such time as it comes in contact with tissues which are cooler. At this point convection once again occurs, except that the heat travels from the blood to the adjacent tissue.

To maintain an internal core temperature of 98.6°F (37°C), the circulatory system transfers heat internally via the blood and moves it to the skin's surface where convection transfers the heat to cooler external tissues. The cooled blood then returns to the internal viscera where it is able to drain off more excess heat and repeat the cycle.

When a large quantity of heat is being generated (either internally or externally), the superficial blood vessels (the ones near the skin's surface) vasodilatate. This action allows more blood to reach the surface, thereby warming the skin tissues. As the pores on the skin open up under the influence of the autonomic nervous system, perspiration can flow, heat is drawn off as a part of the evaporation process, and heat loss is accelerated.

By way of contrast, if the external environment is cold, great amounts of heat would soon be lost if the blood continued to circulate near the skin's surface. To prevent such losses, vasoconstriction occurs: blood flow to the superficial vessels is sharply curtailed (fatty tissue acts as an insulator for them), and heat loss by conduction through the skin is minimized. If vasoconstriction did not occur, the shock of very cold blood returning to the heart from the skin could trigger cardiovascular problems. (By the same token, if a person's core temperature has dropped due to hypothermic conditions, improper rewarming can cause less blood to return to the heart initially, again, there is a risk of cardiovascular complications.)

Vasoconstriction is ultimately one of the body's most effective protective measures in minimizing heat loss. In severely cold conditions, virtually all blood will be shunted away from the extremities which, because of their surface area, are prone to rapid heat loss. The remaining blood passes through such a comparatively large mass of cool tissue that by the time it reaches the outer ends of the hand or foot, the blood will be 15–25°F cooler than the blood in the trunk of the body. Since the quantity of blood circulating in the very cold extremities is so small, heat loss is relatively minor and the blood is thoroughly mixed and warmed by the blood in the trunk before it returns to the heart.

EVAPORATION

The fourth mechanism involved in heat loss is evaporation. Insofar as the human body is concerned, our use of the term *evaporation* will refer to the evaporation of water. Evaporation is a significant mechanism for heat loss because considerable amounts of thermal energy are required to convert water from a liquid to a gaseous state. Water on the skin, for example, continues to absorb thermal energy (via conduction) until such time as the water vaporizes.

Body heat is discharged via the evaporative process in three ways. The first, and perhaps the most commonly perceived, way is as a result of perspiration or sweating. Sweating is an *active* process involving the secretion of fluids (chiefly a weak solution of sodium chloride) by the sweat glands. Those fluids are secreted into ducts which, in turn, lead to pores in the surface of the skin. Overt sweating does not occur continuously, but is instead a periodic reflex controlled by the autonomic nervous system. There are over two million sweat glands in the body and they are capable of producing approximately nine pounds of water *per hour*. When secreted, these fluids are approximately 98.6°F (37°C). Under average temperature and humidity conditions, roughly 2400 kilocalories would be required to vaporize such a quantity of water.

It is important to note that since the fluids are at body temperature when secreted, cooling does not occur unless additional heat is absorbed and unless air temperature and humidity conditions are conducive to evaporation. Relative humidity is probably the most important factor. In air at 100% relative humidity, evaporation does not occur; although the sweat glands may secrete their fluids in an effort to cool the body, the perspiration simply drips off the body and does not serve a cooling function. Thus you may not lose much heat by way of evaporation on hot, muggy days.

When the body is exposed to high environmental temperatures, evaporation plays an increasingly important function. For example, if the ambient air is at 98.6°F (37°C), the same temperature as the body's core and as the skin, heat exchange via radiation or conduction and convection would be negligible, since you need a thermal gradient for radiation, convection or conduction to promote heat transfer. However, since the metabolic furnace is producing heat, the only way for the body to discharge that excess heat is by evaporation. If the ambient temperature is higher than 98.6°F (37°C), then the body will gain heat as a result of radiation, conduction, convection and metabolic action. Here again, evaporation is the only available cooling response; the only response, that is, except for behavioral modification of the environment.

Aside from sweating, two other evaporative processes are at work to help cool the body. One such process is the ongoing diffusion of water through the skin, which is not a completely water-tight covering. This process differs from sweating in that while sweating is an active process controlled by the sympathetic nervous system, diffusion of water occurs simply as a result of the drying of the skin's surface and the movement of moisture through subcutaneous tissues toward the surface. As that moisture reaches the surface of the skin, the body's thermal energy heats the water and the ambient temperature and relative humidity determine the rate of evaporation.

In a similar fashion, moisture moves through the mucous tissues which line the respiratory system. Air movement created by ventilation brings dry air into contact with the moisture and this convection process, as well as the absorption of thermal energy by the water, causes evaporation. The moist water vapor is then discharged as the ventilation process completes its cycle. On the average upward of 600 milliliters of body water per day are evaporated in this way, and a significant amount of body heat is lost as well. The heat loss due to ventilation is somewhat analogous to opening the windows of a house on a cold winter's day to let warmth as well as moisture in the house go outside.

While each of the four heat transfer processes (radiation, conduction, convection and evaporation) account for a considerable portion of heat loss, the processes of evaporation and convection have special relevance to our discussion of hypothermia.

Evaporation is singled out because it has far-reaching consequences, some might call them hidden dangers, when dealing with cold environmental situations. Take, for example, a jogger running on a cold winter morning. The exercise requires a considerable amount of muscular activity. Metabolism must be increased to provide the energy for that activity, and increased metabolism creates a vast quantity of heat which must subsequently be discharged. The heat build-up will be such that the sweat glands will be activated. The sweat glands will secrete their fluids, which will then be vaporized by the body's heat. However, vaporizing that much perspiration requires a considerable caloric output and body temperature is often drained below its optimal level, setting the stage for hypothermia. In addition, the fluid loss associated with the sweating can promote dehydration, which can also make the body more susceptible to hypothermia.

Exercise and subsequent perspiration in cold environments extract great quantities of both heat and moisture from the body. However, in addition to the role of sweating, heat and water vapor are also lost during breathing, the rate of which normally increases during work activity.

To summarize, the following physiological factors will determine the overall net temperature of the body: (1) total metabolic rate; (2) physical work; (3) the rate of evaporative heat loss; and (4) the rate of heat loss or gain by radiation, convection, and conduction.

But physiology and biochemistry do not provide all the answers: the incredible powers of the mind, through the expression of the will to survive, can greatly influence heat production and heat loss. Individual psychology is an important ingredient in survival.

CHAPTER 4

Hypothermia Revisited: What Really Happens

It has been noted that there are many sets of circumstances which can lead to subnormal temperatures. Perhaps the most dramatic and rapid effects are observed when a person is suddenly immersed in very cold water. When the *Titanic* sank in the North Atlantic, her passengers were thrown into water in the range of 0°F (−10°C) and the air temperature was close to that of the water. Many of the passengers were poorly dressed, few had satisfactory life preservers, and all had scant chance for survival. Under such conditions, hypothermia can become a certainty very quickly.

A much different situation faces the backpacker suddenly stranded in the midst of an unexpected early winter blizzard in the mountains. If not well-versed in survival techniques and sufficiently well-dressed, the person may suffer a long painful decline into a state of hypothermia. Body core temperature will drop slowly over a period of several hours, or even for days, but the end result will be similar to that which befell the *Titanic*'s passengers.

These two situations are typical of acute accidental hypothermia, cases in which the onset of hypothermia is relatively sudden and severe.

While hypothermia can arise from a variety of situations, the most clear-cut picture of the effects of subnormal body temperatures can be gained by viewing cases in which there is an acute onset. The progression of hypothermia vividly illustrates the interrelationships between all of the bodily systems which are involved in thermoregulation. Later we will deal with secondary accidental hypothermia, a term used to describe situations in which the drop in body temperature is related to various complicating factors, such as alcohol or cardiovascular problems.

ACUTE HYPOTHERMIA: A PHYSIOLOGICAL OVERVIEW

An individual suffering the effects of acute hypothermia moves through a carefully defined sequence of symptoms, each of which reflects the body's decreased ability to maintain control over its many and varied functions.

There are two major reasons for the lack of scientific certainty regarding the time frame for hypothermia. The first is that the physical condition and the psychological attitude of the victim both serve to accelerate or decelerate the rate of core temperature decline. A physically fit, well-fed person who doesn't panic and who believes he will survive will experience a slower drop in core temperature than someone who is ill-prepared psychologically and physically.

The second reason scientists cannot easily specify the time frame is that the rate of core temperature decline is highly dependent on environmental circumstances. Water at 72°F (22°C) drains body heat faster than water at 81°F (27°C). An air temperature of 54°F (15°C) is bearable if there is no wind and humidity, but with a 25 mph wind and low humidity, that same air can be deadly.

98.6–95°F (37–35°C)—Core Temperature

Regardless of the specific environmental influences, if hypothermic conditions exist the first observable sign is usually shivering. Shivering causes increased metabolic activity which, as we have seen, serves as a warming process.

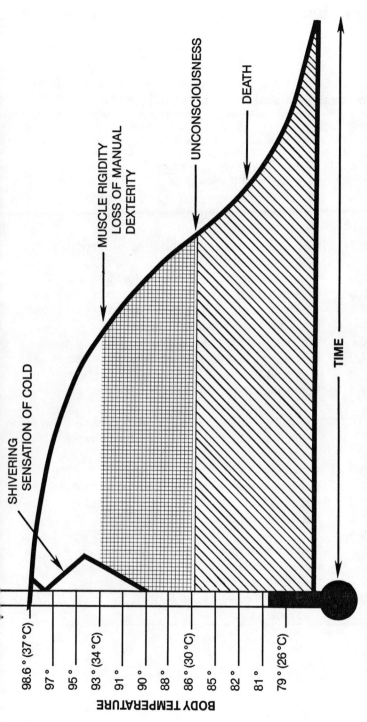

Hypothermia: Because of the wide variations in age, personal reactions, water temperature, and other conditions, no standard measure of time can be applied to the effects of hypothermia on an individual.

Progressive Clinical Presentation of Hypothermia

Core temperature		
°C	°F	Clinical signs
37.6	99.6	"Normal" rectal temperature
37	98.6	"Normal" oral temperature
36	96.8	Metabolic rate increases in an attempt to compensate for heat loss
35	95.0	Maximum shivering
34	93.2	Victim conscious and responsive, with normal blood pressure
33	91.4	Severe hypothermia below this temperature
32 }	89.6 }	Consciousness clouded; blood pressure becomes
31	87.8	difficult to obtain; pupils dialated but react to light; shivering ceases
30 }	86.0 }	Progressive loss of consciousness; muscular
29	84.2	rigidity increases; pulse and blood pressure difficult to obtain; respiratory rate decreases
28	82.4	Ventricular fibrillation possible with myocardial irritability
27	80.6	Voluntary motion ceases; pupils nonreactive to light; deep tendon and superficial reflexes absent
26	78.8	Victim seldom conscious
25	77.0	Ventricular fibrillation may occur spontaneously
24	75.2	Pulmonary edema
22 }	71.6 }	Maximum risk of ventricular fibrillation
21	69.8	
20	68.0	Cardiac standstill
18	64.4	Lowest accidental hypothermia victim to recover
17	62.6	Isoelectric electroencephalogram
9	48.2	Lowest artificially cooled hypothermia patient to recover

This shivering is often triggered by rapid cooling of the skin and serves as a quick, short-term warming function. If the *core* termperature drops below 98.6°F (37°C), shivering always occurs (unless the person is disabled). If shivering fails to restore core temperature to its optimal level, this muscular activity usually ceases once core temperature drops to 90°F (32°C) or below.

Circulation to the outer extremities is typically reduced sharply during the early stages of hypothermia. The skin of the hands and feet, for example, may drop to as low as 40°F (4°C) as a result of environmental factors and reduced blood flow. Despite what seems an extraordinarily low temperature, the tissue often suffers no damage if it is rewarmed properly. But damaged skin or not, sensations of being cold typically dominate a person's consciousness so long as core temperature remains in the 95–98.6°F (35–37°C) range.

Cold air and cold water activate our pain receptors; they cause us to hurt. In and of itself, pain can cause a variety of reactions, among them muscle withdrawal, fear and anger. From a psychological perspective, there are enormous social and cultural differences with respect to the perception of and response to pain. Italian men and Swedish women will react differently to the same pain stimulus; so too will English and Russian men or American men and women. While there have been very few scientific studies conducted on the relationship between these sociocultural factors and fear, cold and pain perception, there is no question among authorities that some people simply can handle cold stress better than others. Psychological preparation is often the critical factor in survival. In situations in which people are being selected for assignments in the cold, the individual's personality is often viewed as being every bit as important as any physiological factor; usually it's considered as being more important. Frequently, very thin people (who theoretically should lose heat quickly) will perform better and last longer in a cold environment than their fatter counterparts (who have more insulation, more metabolic resources, etc.). While higher metabolic rates might work in favor of the thin person, there is much evidence to indicate that "psychic toughness" is really the determining factor. Whether the individual is fat or thin may be a secondary consideration.

Another initial reaction to acute cold stress is increased respiration and ventilation. Rapid breathing, and often hyperventilation, will occur as the body struggles to "fire" its metabolic furnaces. The cold also prompts many people to urinate spontaneously during the early stages of hypothermia.

95–91.4°F (35–33°C)—Core Temperature

Once core temperature drops to this level, consciousness often becomes clouded and the victim will frequently appear dazed and irrational. Restricted blood flow to the limbs as well as altered neuromuscular activity will result in an increasing loss of dexterity. Walking or swimming becomes extremely difficult and control over the hands is often absent. As consciousness continues to decline, speech will become slurred, unusual (sometimes life-threatening) behavior may occur, and the victim may either doze off or wander aimlessly in complete disregard for personal safety.

Psychological withdrawal and complete carelessness appear next; the victim truly no longer cares what happens. From this point on, amnesia may set in, and victims who do recover may never fully recall their experiences.

86–91.4°F (30–33°C)—Core Temperature

Once core temperature drops to the 86–91.4°F (30–33°C) level, several reactions occur. Shivering usually ceases and the muscles become fairly rigid. In many victims, short bursts of random muscular activity will occur, but these violent shudders and shakes do not resemble ordinary shivering, nor do they produce any significant amount of heat. The victim's pupils will dilate, pulse rate will slow down markedly, breathing becomes erratic and shallow, and skin may show some discoloration. Cardiac arrhythmias (irregular disturbances of the normal heart rhythm) frequently are apparent during this stage.

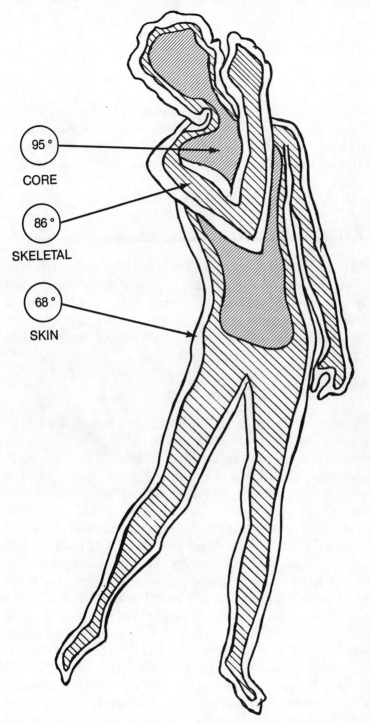

95° CORE

86° SKELETAL

68° SKIN

Even at a core temperature of 95°F, the victim will probably appear dazed and irrational, and walking and swimming will become difficult, often sure signs that hypothermia has seriously begun to take effect.

82.4–86°F (28–30°C)—Core Temperature

Consciousness may lapse completely in this stage or in the next. Deep tendon and skin reflexes will cease and, if additional sudden physical shocks occur, ventricular fibrillation may be triggered. *Ventricular fibrillation* refers to random, totally nonproductive and "convulsive" contractions of the heart muscle which can be lethal.

68–77°F (20–25°C)—Core Temperature

Actually, between 68–77°F (20–25°C), ventricular fibrillation may appear spontaneously and, should this activity continue unchecked, death will occur. The build-up of fluids in the lungs develops at this stage due to changes in the cardiovascular system; these will be discussed later in the chapter.

77°F (25°C)—Core Temperature

For most victims, once core temperature drops to the 77°F (25°C) level, the heart has come to a standstill (asystole), the muscles have become flaccid. Once a victim reaches this point, death is virtually imminent. It should be noted, however, that a hospital patient was successfully revived after core temperature had dropped to 48.2°F (9°C).

As will be noted in a later chapter, successful revival of hypothermia victims has been achieved even though they appeared "dead." Their survival depended on carefully managed, gradual rewarming procedures in which the recovery of each body system was coordinated with that of the others. Since revival is often possible, the rule of thumb for emergency medical and rescue workers is to *use recommended procedures to restore core temperature to 98.6°F (37°C) before pronouncing the victim dead.*

The above-mentioned signs and symptoms obviously result from internal reactions to the progressive decline of core temperature, presumably caused by a major (external) cold stress. We can now examine those reactions in greater detail.

SPECIFIC REACTIONS TO
COLD STRESS 98.6–93.2°F (37–34°C)

The first event in the hypothermia "chain" is that cold air (or water) is sensed by the thermal receptors which are located in the skin or in the respiratory passages of the nose and mouth. These thermal receptors send electrical messages to the brain, warning of the potential threat. If those messages indicate that the body is in danger of losing core heat, the brain orders a series of emergency procedures, including the following.

Vasoconstriction—Peripheral

Initially, if the cold stress is localized (confined to a small area), that site will undergo a vasoconstriction of thensuperficial blood vessels which will divert warm blood elsewhere, usually into the trunk of the body. If heat loss continues, this vasoconstriction process will be extended over a larger and larger area. If the brain has sensed that there is a total body threat (as happens when a person falls into very cold water), widespread vasoconstriction will take place immediately. The victim's skin may suddenly appear chalky as superficial blood vessels in all parts of the body narrow.

Blood Pressure

As vasoconstriction becomes more and more widespread, blood pressure increases because many of the peripheral vessels have constricted their volume, sometimes well in excess of 75%. When reductions in volume of that magnitude occur, either new space must be available for the blood to move into or blood pressure will rise. (The effect is not unlike what happens when you squeeze a water-filled balloon.) Some blood does move into vessels in the internal organs, but the expansion capability is limited and blood pressure is invariably increased.

Epinephrine Release

Simultaneous with the initial vasoconstriction, sensory messages to the brain typically trigger a psychological and physiological "fear" response. This response essentially involves placing the body in a state of preparedness. Epinephrine (adrenaline) as well as various other chemicals produced in the body are released in the blood stream and all body systems are primed for emergency functioning. The most immediate measurable effect of this response is that heart rate increases. Actually, increased heart rate is triggered by two independent mechanisms, neural and hormonal, each serving as a back-up in the event the other should fail for some reason. One set of electrical messages arrives at the heart from the autonomic nervous system. A second set of chemical messages arrives in the form of the hormone epinephrine which, as we have noted, has been released in response to a "stress alert" command from the brain to the adrenal glands. While there is double coverage of this command to increase heart rate, the effect and the function is the same; namely, to circulate oxygen and nutrient-rich blood more rapidly through the system so that muscular tissue will have access to needed metabolic resources should the muscles be called into action.

Cold-Induced Gasping or Acute Respiratory Changes

Another common initial reaction to sudden cold exposure involves a shock to the respiratory system. Simply put, the victim gasps. Most people will gasp at least once, or a few times, but in some individuals this gasping behavior may continue unabated for several minutes. Technically referred to as an *inspiratory arrest,* the sudden exposure to very cold air serves as an unmistakable stimulus to the thermal receptors which line the respiratory tract. In addition, stimulation to cold receptors on the skin by either water or air also contribute to the respiratory arrest. Both sets of receptors send electrical messages to the brain. The brain then initiates a variety of muscular reactions, not the least of which is a momentary increase in ventilation. This new breathing activity increases the supply of oxygen brought into the lungs where respiration (the exchange of oxygen for carbon dioxide) takes place. This increase in ventilation is usually brought under voluntary control within a few gasps.

Overall, these responses can be considered acute:

1. peripheral vasoconstriction;
2. increase in blood pressure;
3. increase in epinephrine release;
4. cold-induced gasping; and
5. increase in heart rate.

Muscle Tension and Shivering

As the internal and external thermal receptors relay their sensory information to the brain, tension within the skeletal muscle system increases rather dramatically. This tension serves two functions. On the one hand, it is a part of the overall preparedness triggered by the perception of stress. On the other hand, muscle tensing increases metabolic activity which results in heat production. In most individuals, muscle tensing will soon be accompanied by overt shivering, the purpose of which has already been discussed. Shivering can continue for long periods of time and is an effective, heat-producing defensive response.

Blood Shunting

As the extremities and limbs become cooler, and as threats to core temperature increase, more and more blood is shunted into the body cavity. This continued shunting of blood is facilitated by vasoconstriction not only of the superficial arteries which service the skin tissue, but by the secondary arteries which serve the muscles and tendons in

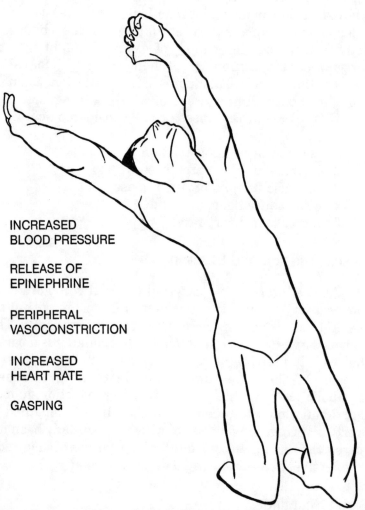

INCREASED
BLOOD PRESSURE

RELEASE OF
EPINEPHRINE

PERIPHERAL
VASOCONSTRICTION

INCREASED
HEART RATE

GASPING

Sudden exposure to sharp cold results in constriction of the blood vessels, gasping for breath, accelerated heart beat, and the release of epinephrine into the blood, causing increased blood pressure.

the limbs. Vasoconstriction of these deep vessels does not usually occur until core temperature has dropped to the vicinity of 89.6–95°F (32–35°C), the point at which shivering ceases. Other symptoms at this stage include a lack of dexterity, increased loss of motor control, and increased rigidity of the muscles.

This rigidity is markedly different from the earlier tensing of muscles. The tensing response helps prepare the body for defensive, survival behaviors and generates heat. The development of muscle rigidity is useful only in that such muscle makes very few demands on the metabolic resources, thus enabling those resources to be used for more critical functions. The rigidity is thought to be caused primarily by a decreased supply of oxygen and glucose for the muscle cells, the build-up of metabolic end products such as carbon dioxide and lactic acid, and altered neuromuscular activity. While this rigid muscle tissue is still "alive and well" and capable of full recovery, it has essentially been shut-down or closed-off (like an unneeded room in a house) so that needed metabolic resources can be used to warm higher priority body parts.

Among those higher priority body parts are the vital organs. Here, as in so many other instances, one must marvel at the efficiency of the body, particularly when viewing responses to hypothermic stress. We noted elsewhere that as vasoconstriction occurs, the blood must be shunted elsewhere. Much of that blood is diverted to the vital organs, thus maintaining and possibly increasing their normal supply of oxygen and nutrients. This diversion of blood to the organs serves a two-fold purpose. Not only does it ensure that heat energy will be available to the organs so that they will be able to continue their lifesaving functions while under severe stress, but it also minimizes heat loss in peripheral areas of the body.

Cold-Induced Diuresis

One specific effect of the diverted blood flow involves the kidneys. The primary function of the kidneys is to filter toxic waste from the blood, and since there is an increased volume of blood flowing through the kidneys (as a result of hypothermic stress), increased quantities of blood are filtered. This filtrate is collected in the bladder, from which it is discharged as urine. Since larger than normal amounts of blood are being processed, people undergoing a cold stress experience increased urine production. This increased urine production naturally flows to the bladder. In addition, the increased volume of blood in the trunk of the body triggers certain blood vessel receptors which are sensitive to changes in blood volume. Those receptors cause the release of several hormones which then promote a voiding of the bladder. This entire process is known as cold-induced diuresis.

BREAKDOWN—95°F (35°C)

As the stress of hypothermia continues, the workload on bodily systems begins to take its toll, and increased breakdowns and alterations of life support functions will occur.

Overall, when the body is no longer able to maintain its temperature at 98.6°F (37°C), there are three ways in which the cold affects each organ system. These three effects center on (1) the individual cells, (2) the hormones that regulate the function of the cells, (3) the nerves that autonomically control the cells and (4) the decrease in oxygen and glucose to the cells.

Brain–Spinal Cord Effects

One such potential breakdown involves behavioral control. Like all cells, those in the brain, our behavioral control center, require glucose for fuel and oxygen. Blood glucose is essential for the proper, coordinated functioning of the nervous system. Since the demands for glucose are quite high under prolonged hypothermic stress, there comes a point at which supplies will be exhausted. While there are many other chemicals involved in brain functions, abnormally low blood glucose levels in the brain can predispose the victim to abnormal, often irrational behavior while conscious. In addition, if oxygen levels are in anyway compromised, the function of the brain will also be compromised.

One example of cold-induced behavior that is "irrational" is a phenomenon known as "paradoxical undressing." For some unexplained reason, many hypothermia victims reach a point at which they begin removing their clothes. Searchers have followed a trail of coats, shoes, shirts, pants, and other garments over long distances, only to find a nude victim at the end. Some victims will undress in one spot and then roll in the snow or on the ground until they lose consciousness.

Other examples of breakdown include a weakening of neural control over skeletal muscles, a drifting in and out of consciousness, and increasing deterioration of autonomic control over cardiac functions. Overall, however, the brain can withstand a great deal of cold stress—at least as long as it is able to obtain oxygen.

As core temperature drops and the vital organs and nervous system are exposed to subnormal levels of cold, every internal function is affected. Clearly, as the nervous system undergoes prolonged exposure to severe cold, the body experiences widespread effects.

We have already noted that the vital organs, and indeed all tissues, experience depressed activity as a result of the decrease in metabolic rate. A second factor which contributes to their reduced functioning is the localized cooling of neural control mechanisms. Each organ, every gland and all other muscle groups are controlled by nerves which ultimately relate to the brain and spinal cord. In addition, most organs and glands have neural reflex loops which provide them with feedback on their own internal functions. In addition to these common reflex loops, most of the major organs, such as the heart and intestinal tract, have what are called nerve plexi imbedded in their structure. These plexi are actually networks of nerves which serve as internal monitoring and control "substations." Each organ's intrinsic plexus is controlled by an external network of nerve cells which communicates more directly with the brain and spinal cord. The advantage of these imbedded networks is that the major organs have semi-independent systems of neural control which help promote functioning.

Nonetheless, the effects of cold eventually do make themselves known to the organs. When the nerve cells that comprise these control networks, reflex loops and plexi are chilled, the efficiency and speed with which they operate are reduced. From a completely hypothetical perspective, even if the organs were receiving their normal blood supply and if metabolism were also normal, bodily systems would be slowed simply as a result of the cooling of the nerve cells. Neural functioning is affected by the cold in two ways and, as we have noted, this impaired functioning ultimately affects every other organ, muscle and cell in the body.

The first way that nerve cells are affected relates to the way in which nerve cells "communicate" with other cells (such as those in the heart or arterial tissue). This communication occurs primarily as a result of electrical signals which are transferred from cell to cell. These minute signals run from cell to cell like dominos falling, jumping from cell to cell until the brain (or heart or artery) is reached.

What happens in hypothermic situations is that the metabolism of the cell is decreased and it becomes increasingly difficult for electrical signals to be exchanged between nerve cells and our muscles, organs, glands, etc. The generation of an electrical signal is not stopped by the cold: the rate of reaction has simply been slowed to the body's equivalent of a "snail's pace." As long as oxygen is available and as long as the cells have not been physically damaged, they will continue to function, albeit at a very slow level of activity.

While the preceding paragraphs relate to the cold-induced slowing down of reactions between nerve cells and muscle cells, the cold also affects the relationship between nerve cells themselves. Although they are highly specialized, nerve cells are like all other cells in that they have their own metabolic processes. Just as cold affects the activity of other cells, so too will it slow down the metabolic rate of nerve cells. As that rate declines, the cells can no longer function as efficiently or as quickly as they do under normal circumstances. This metabolic slow-down affects everything from eye–hand coordination to heartbeat and vascular control. It simply takes longer for the nerve cells to transmit or respond to neural messages.

One final observation should be made concerning the nervous system. There are a number of physiological behaviors or actions which are technically termed *reflex responses*. The common knee-jerk response is an example; so too is the response the pupil makes to different intensities of light. There are many other possible examples, some of which include actions by our glands and organs.

In any event, these responses are governed by well-defined neural feedback loops. Each such response is rapid and does not require any involvement or "decision" by the brain. Characteristically, certain reflex responses are initially excited by cold exposure. This excitement is undoubtedly related to the body's initial pattern of response to stress. The reflex responses are simply a way of placing the body in a state of heightened sensitivity, preparing it for protective action. Between the temperatures of 98.6°F (37°C) and 86°F (30°C) such reflex responses as shivering, pupillary dilation and pain are especially sensitive and active. Once core temperature drops below 86°F (30°C), however, those reflexes are sharply depressed since the electrical signals are traveling slower and their response time is delayed significantly. *Since this pattern is well established, you can use reflex behaviors as a rough guide to core temperature. A hypothermia victim who is shivering almost certainly has a core temperature above 86°F (30°C). On the other hand, a victim who is not shivering, who shows no response to pain and whose pupils do not respond to changes in light almost certainly has a core temperature below 86°F (30°C).*

Cardiovascular System

We can also observe major impacts from the cold on the circulatory system. Recall that initially the circulatory system experienced an increase in both heart rate and blood pressure. But after prolonged exposure, the heart muscle and the nerves which control it are chilled. In addition to lowered metabolic activity, this physical chilling of the heart and neural tissue results in an increasingly slower heart rate. This rate may eventually drop off to one or two contractions a minute.

Interestingly, although the heartbeat slows markedly, the heart itself increases in efficiency. This increase occurs because during the period when the heart is not contracting, a larger than normal quantity of blood flows into its chambers, distending it beyond its normal size. One characteristic of the heart is that the greater the volume of blood in the chambers, the more powerful will be the contraction created to expel that blood. Thus, under hypothermic conditions, 2–3 heartbeats per minute may be completely adequate for circulating blood throughout the metabolically decreased system.

For the person in normal physiological health, the thought of 2–3 heartbeats per minute is terrifying—hence the tendency for inexperienced rescue parties to rush in and start pounding on a hypothermia victim's chest. Cardiac functions are among the last to fail in hypothermia victims, regardless of external signs, or lack thereof.

Understanding that the heart can function quite efficiently at low temperatures is absolutely essential for anyone who may be faced with rescue or treatment of hypothermia victims. Under such conditions, a very slow powerful heartbeat is entirely normal. *No effort should be made to increase heart rate using such techniques as external chest compression.*

Chest compressions administered to the hypothermia victim at this point can be lethal because they will, in all likelihood, reduce the efficiency of the heart and they may cause ventricular fibrillation.

Remember that when it is very cold, the heart is filling with a large quantity of blood between contractions. All that blood will be adequately distributed by the heart when it contracts. The chest compression (or any blow to the victim's chest) causes a premature, artificial contraction of the heart muscle and thus sends an inadequate amount of blood into the arteries.

Equally important is the fact that when the heart tissue and its neural network are physically cold, they are highly susceptible to mechanical disturbances. In a sense, they aren't prepared to handle the stress of physical abuse. The nerves can't control the muscle reactions created by chest compressions, and there is thus a strong possibility that ventricular fibrillation will set in.

Ventricular fibrillation is an unsynchronized muscular contraction of the heart. Instead of a coordinated contracting of the four chambers of the heart, individual muscle cells relax and contract randomly. This behavior on the part of the heart is lethal since virtually no blood is moved out of the heart and an extraordinary amount of oxygen and glucose is consumed by the heart muscles as they fibrillate. Unless corrected immediately, this condition can be fatal.

The subject of ventricular fibrillation relates to yet another very important point concerning hypothermia and its impact on people, such as athletes or hypertensive individuals, who have enlarged hearts. All hearts, whether normal or enlarged, have a very specific electrical pattern which is governed by the intrinsic and extrinsic neural systems described earlier. This pattern includes an instant during which the nervous system fires a command and an instant in which the nerve cells which control the heart are "recharging" themselves. The time span during which this recharging is occurring is called a period of hyperexcitability. What this implies is that since the nerve cells are busy recharging, they are not really in a position to coordinate the heart muscle activity. Until the recharging is completed, the heart muscle is particulary susceptible to random or irregular (unexpected) electrical signals.

Everyone's heart has a period of hyperexcitability, and this period increases in cold temperatures. What is important is that when cold, the enlarged heart seems to develop a proportionately longer period of hyperexcitability. The reason that this is of concern with respect to hypothermia victims is that many hypothermic situations start with a sudden shock—such as falling into a cold mountain stream. Sudden shocks trigger immediate electrical messages and chemical (epinephrine) messages to the heart; those messages command increased heart beat and increased blood pressure. The heart must be able to respond at an appropriate point in its cycle. If those messages arrive during the period of hyperexcitability, there is a significant likelihood that a deviate response will occur: that is, cardiac arrhythmia or ventricular fibrillation may be triggered. Thus, for the person with an enlarged heart, the danger of a sudden cold shock may not lie so much with hypothermia, but rather from the shock and its implications for cardiac functioning. In many of the cases reported each year of people who fell into cold water and then died minutes later, there is good reason to believe that death was brought on not by hypothermia, but by acute cardiac problems associated with this period of hyperexcitability.

There are also several other cardiovascular implications arising from the effects of cold. Within the system as a whole, there is a decrease in blood pressure because the heart is not beating very often. Because a great deal of blood has been shunted into the core areas, the blood vessels are engorged with blood, although it's not moving very rapidly. The slow movement of the blood (due to relatively infrequent heart beats) is further decreased by the increasing viscosity of the blood. So sensitive is the blood to cold temperatures that for every 1°C drop in temperature, there is a 1% increase in its viscosity. While this increase in viscosity seems small, even a moderate increase in the "thickness" of the blood causes the heart to work much harder. Increased viscosity also complicates circulation in the capillaries throughout the body.

Aside from its heat-distribution function, the primary purpose of the blood is to transport oxygen to the cells. This critical function involves hemoglobin, a chemical compound in the blood, which picks up oxygen in the lungs. Hemoglobin transports oxygen to the individual cells where it delivers the oxygen and picks up carbon dioxide, a by-product of metabolism. The carbon dioxide is then returned to the lungs from whence it is expelled.

Since metabolism is occuring *very slowly* in this "metabolic icebox," as we might call the hypothermia victim, very little carbon dioxide is being produced and very little oxygen is required. Because of this sharp reduction in metabolic activity, many persons have been able to survive severe hypothermic situations. The cold so drastically reduces metabolic activity that even a nominal amount of oxygen in the blood is often able to sustain life.

Ventilation–Respiration

It is perhaps because the body's oxygen requirements are so low in the hypothermic state that breathing activity is the first of the "vital signs" to (apparently) cease. In fact, ventilation, the movement of air into and out of the lungs, acts like all of the body's other systems in severe cold, it slows down to the point of being barely perceptible. Metabolic activity in the body can become so slow that one breath every 30 seconds or so may be all the body needs; with so little breathing required, vital signs are very difficult to detect in hypothermia victims. Ultimately, of course, ventilation will cease entirely. Interestingly, after that last gasping breath, there may still be enough oxygen in the circulatory system of the hypothermia victim to sustain him or her for a prolonged period of time. This is due to the fact that hemoglobin in the blood will hold the oxygen until it is needed by the cells. What we usually think of as breathing is comprised of three separate, but highly interrelated systems: ventilation, respiration and circulation.

Ventilation is the term used to refer to the actual process of moving air into and out of the lungs. The muscles of the chest wall and the diaphragm are responsible for the movement; the operating principle is no different from that of an ordinary fireplace bellows.

Inside the lungs, the bronchial tubes subdivide into

secondary and tertiary bronchi, ending in many bronchiole and alveolar ducts. At the end of each such duct are the alveoli themselves. The *alveoli* are tiny balloon-like airpockets. The alveolar walls are extremely thin membranes. These tiny pockets fill with air during inhalations. The oxygen in the air is selectively allowed to pass through the membranes where the oxygen molecules attach themselves to blood hemoglobin that is accessible in the tiny alveolar capillaries which line the outside of the pocket. At the same time that oxygen is attaching itself to the hemoglobin, carbon dioxide (a metabolic by-product) is being kicked off the hemoglobin molecule and is passing through the membranes in the other direction: it enters the pocket where it is discharged during exhalation. This oxygen–carbon dioxide transfer process is called *respiration*.

Circulation is critical to this process since the alveoli must be perfused with red blood cells, which have the hemoglobin, and are the only ones which can carry out the oxygen transport and the oxygen–carbon dioxide exchange processes. Once the blood has picked up fresh oxygen, it returns to the heart via the pulmonary veins; from the heart the blood is pumped out to serve the body tissues. Once the oxygen has been delivered to the cells, carbon dioxide is picked up, returned to the lungs (via the heart), and the cycle repeats itself.

All three of these intertwined processes (ventilation, respiration and circulation) are coordinated in both normal and hypothermia situations. In many victims, ventilation is the first of the three components to fail, but as noted, the victim may still be alive (and revivable). Respiration and circulation may continue long after ventilation has ceased.

Like the other systems we have examined, the ventilation and respiratory processes are gradually suppressed by prolonged exposure to the cold. Typically ventilation, respiration and circulation will continue until core temperature drops to the vicinity of 20°C. Well above that level, however, ventilation may have become so infrequent as to be judged absent. Rescue workers must make every effort to determine

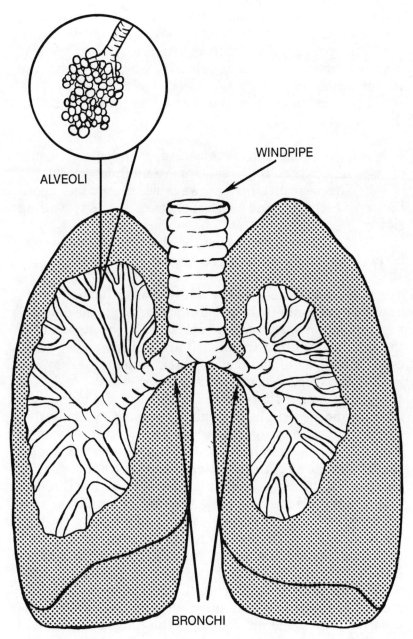

ALVEOLI

WINDPIPE

BRONCHI

The lungs, including windpipe, bronchi, and the tiny air pockets within the bronchi, known as alveoli.

if the victim is ventilating at all. If ventilation is present, one must assume that the heart is beating. Even if ventilation is not present, the circulatory and respiratory systems may be functioning; although clearly, survival time for the victim is limited.

The slowing down of the ventilation process is due to three factors:

1. The entire body has cooled, metabolism is suppressed and oxygen requirements are minimal.

2. The neural reflex pathways which regulate ventilation are chilled and control messages are travelling slowly.

3. As the body gets colder the chest walls and muscles become more difficult to move.

Once ventilation does actually cease, the next major complication to affect the respiratory system is the development of "pulmonary edema." Recall that the structure of the lung is such that the alveoli are served by very small capillaries. One of the major consequences of severe cold is that the blood becomes increasingly viscous, and as it does, it no longer flows as easily through the pulmonary arteries and, especially, through the pulmonary capillaries. The thick, slow-moving blood which does make its way as far as the capillaries serving the alveoli is so abnormal that it causes a swelling of the alveolar tissue and that distension makes it all the more difficult for the blood to flow through. Eventually, this building pressure causes plasma (the noncellular fluid which makes blood "liquid") to seep through the capillary walls and to fill the alveolar cavities. This is called pulmonary edema. As the fluid builds, it becomes increasingly difficult for the oxygen exchange to occur. (Under normal circumstances, the development of pulmonary edema is first noticeable because it causes "shortness of breath.") This build-up of fluid in the lungs as a result of circulatory problems in the hypothermia victim further compromises what was at best a marginal exchange of oxygen and carbon dioxide. As ventilation ceases and existing oxygen supplies are used up, the victim moves into a state of *hypoxia*, the depletion of oxygen in the body's cells. Once the supply is fully depleted, death is unavoidable.

While hypothermic affects on the body's three major systems (circulatory, nervous, and respiratory) are among the more dramatic and critical, virtually every organ and system is also affected sooner or later by the advancing cold.

With respect to the gastrointestinal tract, for example, hypothermia at even moderate levels, say those in which core temperature is hovering around the 93.2°F (34°C) mark, reduces the function of the stomach and causes a reduction in the quantity of the gastrointestinal secretions. Since the major function of this particular system is to secrete the fluids which initiate the biochemical digestion of foodstuffs into metabolically usable resources and to move the digested bulk through the intestines, the effect of hypothermia is comparable to that of a clamp on the system. Individuals who become even slightly hypothermic frequently experience constipation problems, lasting for several days, due to the effects of the cold. Obviously, this interference in digestion, and hence metabolism, makes it difficult for the victim to replenish dwindling resources; for the victim who has been rescued, time will be required before he or she will be able to return to a normal diet.

A particularly critical shutdown occurs when the cold finally affects the pancreas. The pancreas, as noted, is responsible for the production and secretion of insulin as well as other chemical hormones involved in glucose regulation. Insulin is absolutely essential in the human body; its function is to facilitate the transport of glucose across the membranes of all cells. Without insulin, the cells of the body are deprived of their energy source. As if that weren't bad enough, when the nervous system is deprived of glucose, disorientation, convulsions, unconsciousness and death result.

Hypothermic impact on the liver is an important consideration not only because of immediate effects on the "normal" hypothermia victim, but because of its implications for those who may have ingested alcohol or some other chemical substance. The main function of the liver is to detoxify the blood by neutralizing those metabolic end products which make their way into the bloodstream. Even though the liver, like all other organs, initially experiences increased blood flow during the early stages of hypothermia, blood flow decreases as hypothermia progresses; consequently this organ also experiences a depressed level of functioning over a period of time. Its major blood purifying function is limited and as a consequence, the toxic substances remain chemically active in the bloodstream much longer that they would under normal circumstances.

Ultimately, of course, the cold slows down all of the body's processes until they can no longer support life. Depending on the individual's health status and physical condition, some organ systems will fail sooner than others, but once the respiratory, circulatory or neural systems fail, death comes quickly.

CHAPTER 5

Secondary Accidental Hypothermia

In our examination of *primary* accidental hypothermia we saw how prolonged exposure to low temperature can cause the breakdown of various body systems which, if left unchecked, can lead eventually to permanent organ damage or death. The critical factor in all of this is that those breakdowns and the body's malfunctioning are the *consequences* of primary accidental hypothermia.

In *secondary* accidental hypothermia, the concern is with various diseases or drug-induced disorders which cause the body to malfunction and thus *predispose* the individual to hypothermia. In some cases, various bodily problems which have existed prior to any particular environmental stress can compromise the individual's ability to withstand stress, thus placing the person at a distinct disadvantage.

The development of hypothermia that is directly or indirectly associated with the malfunctioning of one or more of the body's systems can occur in one of three major ways. First, there may be complications which detract from the body's ability to produce heat. Second, there can be complications which contribute to increased heat loss. Third, there may be an interference with the neural mechanisms responsible for thermoregulation. The nervous system plays a central role in almost all these complications, particularly those associated with drugs and medications.

69

The nervous system which controls the body, as well as all our thermoregulatory functions, is comprised of a vast network of nerve cells. These cells activate our muscles, glands and organs, as well as perform in a wide variety of other functions. To perform their duties, nerve cells communicate with each other via chemical secretions. Small quantities of chemicals (called neurotransmitters) are secreted by the nerve cell; the neurotransmitter comes in contact with specific receptor sites on an adjoining nerve cell and "excite" (or inhibit) it. The neurotransmitter is then drawn back into its original cell. If a cell is excited it will secrete a neurotransmitter to its adjoining cell(s). In order for the brain, and the rest of the nervous system, to function correctly, the proper function of a certain number of neurotransmitters must be maintained at all times. Any disturbance of those neurotransmitters by other chemicals, injuries or other external influences will adversely affect neural functioning.

DRUG-INDUCED HYPOTHERMIA

Alcohol (ethanol) figures in hypothermia in several ways, chiefly because of its effects on the central nervous system. For example, it causes a decrease of blood glucose so there is less energy available for cellular metabolism; it depresses higher brain functions (thereby affecting behavor reaction time and thermoregulation), it causes an inappropriate vasodilatation (inappropriate insofar as the potential impact of the cold is concerned) and it causes a "numbing" or desensitization of the thermal receptors.

Alcohol is but one of many drugs used with or without a prescription which significantly alter the thermoregulatory processes. It is not uncommon for drugs to so drastically alter a person's thermoregulatory processes that even a slight thermal stress will trigger the onset of severe hypothermia. In addition to alcohol, the phenothiazines, the barbiturates, and general anesthetics are the one most likely to establish these conditions.

Alcohol consumption can lead to heat loss almost immediately. Once ethanol is ingested, it enters the bloodstream very quickly, prompting vasodilatation, especially of the superficial blood vessels. This vasodilatation causes flushed skin and the impression of being warm, but in cold environments, it promotes rapid heat loss. In many persons ethanol reduces, or even eliminates, the shivering response, thus removing an important heat generating activity as well as an important signal that "all is not right" with the victim's thermal balance. It is also believed that ethanol depresses the thermoregulatory control center, thus reducing the effectiveness of the early warning signs and of the other, more critical, cold stress response mechanisms. Alcohol also reduces blood glucose in some people, our primary fuel for heat production. For some individuals in cold environments, alcohol causes a significant drop in core temperature; this occurs in addition to its other effects on the thermoregulation.

Chronic alcoholics often have severe liver damage which can affect their metabolic processes. It is suspected that many alcoholics have also suffered irreparable damage to the hypothalamus, which, as noted earlier, is critical to the effective functioning of the body's thermoregulatory control processes.

Yet another problem associated with ethanol is behavioral. If quantities of alcohol sufficient to cause intoxication have been ingested, irresponsible actions and poor judgment are often the result. The individual may inadvertently place himself in dangerous situations where the threat of severe exposure exists, or he may simply fail to take reasonable protective measures. Stepping out for a "breath of fresh air" in the middle of winter while wearing nothing more than ordinary indoor clothing has left many an intoxicated person hypothermic in a snowbank.

The way that alcohol affects the human body varies greatly from person to person. Studies have shown that intoxicated persons who are standing still in a cold environment do not lose heat any faster than nonintoxicated persons, but the differential heat loss may be related to drinking history and to the other systemic effects of alcohol on the body. One thing is certain, most intoxicated persons do not behave in their own best interest when in life-threatening situations. Significantly, the vast majority of hospital hypothermia cases involve persons who have consumed excessive quantities of alcohol.

PHENOTHIAZINES

Phenothiazines are drugs usually prescribed in the treatment of depression. Their effect on thermoregulation is particularly unique in that they often cause a person to become hypothermic in cold environments and hyperthermic in hot environments. Several anecdotal cases have been reported in which persons being treated with phenothiazines attempted to commit suicide by jumping into cold water. Rescue attempts were made only to discover that the person's core temperature has been set at a lower temperature. Instead of being at 98.6°F (37°C), the drug has apparently lowered it to 95°F (35°C). The victim was thus saved by the relatively delayed response to the cold stress caused by the drug.

The specific impact of the phenothiazines is not well-understood, but it is clearly apparent that they make a person much more susceptible to both hypothermia and hyperthermia.

BARBITURATES

Barbiturates are used primarily as tranquilizers and are known to induce hypothermia on their own. A deadly combination arises when persons mix alcohol with barbiturates and then are exposed to cold stress. The two drugs augment each other's hypothermia-inducing properties and can kill very quickly.

GENERAL ANESTHETICS

General anesthetics usually depress the entire central nervous system, including the thermoregulatory centers. A number of cases of hypothermia have been reported in which the patient entered a hypothermic state while under the anesthetic.

MARIJUANA (Tetrahydrocannibis)

Marijuana has been reported to cause hypothermia. Although relatively few scientific studies have been made concerning marijuana-induced hypothermia, the present consensus is that it causes an increased sensitivity to cold so that the victim shivers sooner and, more importantly fatigues sooner, which promotes an accelerated drop in core temperature. It may create these effects by influencing the excitability of the neurons involved in the thermoregulatory system. An equally important problem can arise when sensory awareness is dampened and users place themselves in potentially dangerous situations. Heroin intoxication has also been associated with hypothermia in several instances.

PROPRANOLOL

Propranolol and certain other drugs used in treating high blood pressure have been implicated in hypothermia cases. The majority of these medications alleviate hypertension by action on the autonomic nervous system and have the potential for interfering with thermoregulation.

LITHIUM

Lithium, a drug used in treating neurological and psychological disorders, has a definite effect on the brain, apparently by altering neurotransmitter release. The thermoregulatory centers are among the areas affected, and persons who are on lithium therapy run a higher than normal risk of hypothermia when exposed to cold temperatures for prolonged periods.

HYPOTHERMIA AND DRUG ADMINISTRATION

One must exercise great caution whenever a drug is given to a hypothermic victim because severe and often unexpected medical complications can suddenly arise. It will be recalled that in the hypothermic state, metabolism has slowed down, as have the functions of key organs, particularly the kidneys and the liver. These organs, especially the liver, are involved in the breakdown of various drugs. To the extent that liver function is impaired by hypothermia, the drug will remain active in the system longer. If rewarming is undertaken in absence of medical supervision, chemical substances in the bloodstream can suddenly become quite active and have a disasterous impact on what might have otherwise been a normal recovery for the hypothermia victim. For example, in an emergency situation, a rescuer might administer an injection of insulin (a common technique in certain types of emergencies) only to find no observable effect. If a second injection is then given and the victim is subsequently warmed, this double dose of insulin could cause a severe depletion of blood glucose which could lead to brain dysfunction. It is important to remember that the hypothermic state is not a normal state and the effects of any agent given to the hypothermia victim must be constantly monitored.

DISEASES AND DISORDERS THAT MAY INDUCE HYPOTHERMIA

Any traumatic event or disease which affects the metabolic process will alter heat production since it is only through metabolism that the body can generate its own heat. Other health problems can accelerate heat loss or interfere with the body's thermoregulatory process.

Chief among the diseases which contribute to decreased

heat production and to the development of hypothermia are those involving the endocrine system. In conjunction with the nervous system, the endocrine system provides one of our body's most important communications network. The endocrine glands secrete hormones which are chemical messengers, traveling throughout the body via the circulatory system. There are approximately three dozen major different hormones in the body and these chemical messengers are so sophisticated that they can carry commands to specific target cells, thereby activating a particular organ or gland. Since every organ involved in the thermoregulatory system is dependent upon hormones at one level or another, endocrine disorders can severely affect our ability to maintain an appropriate core temperature.

One of the most commonly encountered diseases of this type is severe hypothyroidism (technically called myxedema). This disease, which is most often found in women, involves insufficient production of one of the thyroid's hormones. Lack of this hormone severely depresses metabolic heat production and victims of the disease always feel cold, even when in a moderately warm room.

While the disease can cause a wide range of problems, certain people can have it for months, or even years, without actually developing hypothermia. Eventually, however, about 80% of all hypothyroid victims will develop some degree of hypothermia. In many, if not most, cases exposure to severe cold can bring on a comatose state very quickly. Prior to becoming comatose, victims will often appear to be confused or to be in a stupor; some will exhibit severe personality disorders. Eventually, cardiac failure, pulmonary edema and renal failure occur as complications of the hypothermic coma.

Hypopituitarism (abnormal pituitary function) is associated with hypothermia in the same way that severe hypothyroidism is. The pituitary gland, in conjunction with the hypothalamus, is involved in regulating the thyroid gland, among other functions. Thus, when the pituitary gland is itself functioning at subnormal levels, the thyroid cannot function properly either. If the adrenal gland is altered in terms of function, then hypothermia can also occur since the gland secretes epinephrine (adrenalin).

Hypoglycemia is a disorder characterized by abnormally low levels of blood sugar (glucose). The condition can result from a number of causes, many of them involving one or more of the endocrine glands. Many diabetics who are unable to properly regulate their blood glucose level give themselves more insulin than is necessary in an attempt to remain "energized." The insulin accelerates the transport of glucose across the cell wall membranes. As one might expect, the glucose is metabolized, thus producing excess heat. Initially, the victim will feel flushed and sweat profusely, but once the glucose has been metabolized in this inefficient, rapid-fire manner, the body's resources are markedly reduced, thus lowering the victim's capability to respond quickly and effectively to cold stress.

A further, and more serious, complication arises from the fact that hypoglycemia often affects the central nervous system and the hypothalamus, which is thought to serve as a "coordinator" of the other neural regulatory centers and thus plays a central role in thermoregulation. As the central nervous system and especially the hypothalamus become affected in the progression of hypoglycemia, the metabolic process often malfunctions, thus severely reducing the body's ability to generate heat.

"Insulin-induced" hypoglycemia develops *very rapidly,* and its victims often pass out. Since the body has very little glucose in its blood, the unconscious victim can rapidly become hypothermic.

Shivering, it will be recalled, is an important mechanism for metabolic heat production. Once the brain "decides" that the peripheral temperature is too low or is dropping too fast, we have no control over the shiver reflex.

Any disease, such as a muscular dystrophy, which affects the body's network of muscles, will reduce the individual's ability to shiver. Among the elderly, one very often sees a reduction in body muscle as a concomitant of disease or aging. This reduced muscle mass also reduces the effectiveness of shivering. Then too, among many older persons, the neuromuscular control network for shivering is impaired and effective shivering will simply not occur, even though the person might feel quite cold.

Among the sick, the disabled and the elderly, disease, boredom and neglect often contribute to chronic inactivity. It will be recalled that bodily activity requires muscle movement and that such movement increases metabolic activity and heat. With increased metabolism, heat is produced and the potential for hypothermia is lessened. Persons confined to bed or to a wheelchair because of broken bones, strokes, paralysis of one type or another, arthritis or various other crippling disabilities are particularly prone to hypothermia simply because of their inactivity.

Others for whom inactivity can lead to hypothermic problems include the obese, vagrants (who are usually ill-clothed and poorly sheltered) and victims of violent crimes, such as assault. Elderly persons who fall, in their homes or outside, are often unable to regain their footing and so they lie helpless and susceptible to chilling.

Like fatty tissue, the skin also serves an extremely important insulating function for the body. Diseases which affect the skin in any significant way can have a dramatic effect on the insulating characteristics of the body's durable, but not inviolate covering.

For example, psoriasis and exfoliative dermatitis are two skin diseases which involve an increased amount of peripheral blood flow. The consequence of this increased blood flow is accelerated heat loss. These diseases also affect the skin's ability to diffuse excess moisture and to evaporate sweat.

Still another very serious predisposing hazard lies with the burn victim. Burns affect the skin's protection from the cold, its passive diffusion and evaporative functions, and its detection of cold stimuli. When there is damage to large areas of the epidermis and, especially, of the underlying muscle and connective tissue, the body's ability to restrict heat loss is severely compromised. Damage to these tissues often renders the affected portion of the anatomy completely ineffective with respect to the entire thermoregulatory process. All caution must be exercised with burn victims to protect them from the cold and from unnecessary heat loss. When severe burns affecting significant areas of the body are involved, the traditional warning signs of hypothermia cannot be expected to occur.

Surprisingly, some people are actually allergic to the cold. When subjected to cold shocks, they will break out in hives and their skin will itch continuously. The reaction can be so severe as to cause shock. In some victims of this disease, air conditioning, swimming or even cold milk shakes can precipitate an attack. In this latter case, the resulting hives inside the throat have been known to cause asphixiation and death.

Cerebral disorders of many types can affect the brain, the spinal cord and the hypothalamus, located deep in the center of the head at the brainstem. In general, any trauma to the head, neck or spinal cord has potential for affecting the body's thermoregulatory functions. Any accident in which there is a blow to the head, neck or spinal cord will likely involve some impairment of thermoregulatory capability; at the very least, there is a strong potential for such impairment. Accident victims must be watched closely. Typically, when there is injury to the spinal cord, victims will lose their thermoregulatory capability for all portions of their body lying below the point of injury. Individuals injured in situations where cold exposure is likely must be protected since the body's normal thermoregulatory processes may not be working and they may not be able to sense cold in certain parts of the body. Persons who have suffered a blow to either the brain or spinal cord may very well have an impaired capability for shivering.

Degenerative diseases of nervous tissue, such as multiple sclerosis, can also seriously affect neural functioning and thus interfere with thermoregulation.

A wide range of circulatory problems can influence brain activity. Cerebral hemmorhaging and strokes, subdural hematoma (abnormal "pockets" of blood in the brain), and any of a number of intracranial lesions can so drastically alter normal nervous activity that thermoregulation is disrupted.

Paraplegics and quadraplegics must be very cautious when in cold environments since below the site of the injury to their spinal cord their circulatory and nervous systems cannot respond adequately to thermal stress.

For persons experiencing many diseases, a depressed level of metabolic activity and heat production is common; it is simply a part of the normal disease process, particularly with viral infections. Bacterial infections (such as those associated with streptococcus) can often affect the brain and the nervous system. When this occurs, there may be thermoregulatory problems resulting in impaired heat production or accelerated heat loss.

STARVATION AND MALNUTRITION

Starvation and malnutrition are conditions which have an obvious association with hypothermia. If an individual is consuming an inadequate or insufficient diet, his cells will not have enough protein, carbohydrates or lipids. As a consequence, cellular metabolism will be inadequate for normal body functions, let alone for the stress of severe cold.

Starvation and malnutrition also contribute to other disorders and conditions which weaken the victim's resistance. Depending on the specific way that starvation and malnutrition manifest themselves in a given individual, there could be cardiovascular, respiratory or nervous system involvement. To the extent that any one of these systems is compromised, so too will the victim be in danger of falling prey to hypothermia.

Starvation and malnutrition are found most frequently among the poor and the elderly, but even many middle- and upper-income children and adults live on nutritionally marginal (poorly balanced) diets. With reference to the elderly, it is worthwhile noting that many older people have gastrointestinal problems or diseases, such as severe anemia, which can indirectly affect their nutritional status, thus predisposing them to hypothermia.

Malnutrition also occurs frequently among people who work or play in unusually cold outdoor conditions. Examples would include backpackers, mountain climbers, scuba and deep-sea divers, military personnel, and construction workers. Often, prolonged dependence on "trail" rations provides such people with only marginal food resources, thus creating an unexpected condition of malnourishment. The stage is then set for the rapid onset of hypothermia.

Malnutrition is a double-edged sword. On the one hand, it deprives the individual of metabolic (heat generating) resources; it can also serve to reduce or nearly eliminate subcutaneous fat, which serves an important insulating function. The person whose subcutaneous fat layers are inadequate will experience more rapid heat loss than will someone whose diet has sustained a healthy layer of such fatty tissue. Persons suffering from anorexia nervosa provide a vivid illustration of this point.

The physiological effects of malnutrition and starvation are often so pronounced that they can cause persons in the tropical zones to develop hypothermia. This may seem paradoxical, but it is typical of secondary accidental hypothermia. *Many of the drugs, diseases, and disorders which can predispose a person to hypothermia are so powerful that they often cause hypothermia in situations where there is no apparent thermal stress.* Many hypothermia victims have been found in the middle of summer in warm climates. Had their bodies been functioning normally, hypothermia would not have been a problem. However, drug or other disease involvement so drastically altered their thermoregulatory mechanism that hypothermia was induced.

CHAPTER 6

SPECIAL CONSIDERATIONS IN HYPOTHERMIA

WORK AND RECREATION IN THE COLD

Jogging outdoors in the winter poses certain problems with respect to thermal regulation, as do many other types of outdoor sports such as skiing, ice-skating, camping, hunting, hiking and mountaineering, and occupations such as ranching, petroleum research work and construction, and while the following comments use a jogger running in cold temperatures as an example, the same physical principles apply to all persons working or exercising in cold temperatures or chilling conditions. Many factors enter into the body's response to physical exertion in cold weather, and the assumption will be made here that the person in question is in good physical health and has become accustomed to the type of work or exercise being performed.

Running generates a tremendous amount of heat due to the fact that much physical work is being performed by various muscle groups. The heat created warms the entire body and, as it does, the temperature of the skin increases. As skin and muscle temperature rises, thermal receptors notify the nervous system of this increase in heat and the brain causes the superficial blood vessels to dilate. This vasodilatation allows the blood to cool. If the superficial blood flow is not sufficient to cool the blood before it returns to the core, perspiration will be initiated as a second cooling response. Ventilation will also increase and, as it does more oxygen is brought into the body to assist in metabolism, and additional body heat is expelled through the mouth and nose. All of this muscular activity as well as the cooling processes require a considerable amount of energy, so that the body's reserves of glucose are consumed at a fairly rapid rate.

Some specific points to consider are these:

1. As a person runs in cold weather, he or she creates a wind *effect* which, combined with whatever wind may be occurring naturally, drains heat from all parts of the body. The rate at which heat is thus removed depends not only on the combined air speed, but on the thermal difference between runner and environment. If the runner is out on a 30°F (−1.1°C) day and the body's core temperature is 98.6°F (37°C), there will be a significant heat loss. If the wind itself is moving at seven miles per hour, the environmental temperature is, in effect, equivalent to 20°F (−6.6°C), and if the runner is moving at a speed of five miles per hour, the equivalent air temperature is, in effect, approximately 10°F (−12.2°C). Under these conditions, there is, in effect, almost a 90° temperature difference between body and environment; such a difference can account for a great heat loss.

2. Although it is usually offset by air speed and other factors, some heat gain may result from the radiant heat reflected by an existing snow cover.

3. Regardless of air temperature, if the amount of excess heat generated is equal to that offset by wind and temperature, no sweating will occur and, as long as the runner has sufficient energy reserves, he or she will be fine. If the runner is wearing clothing which insulates the body from the environment, then heat loss will be diminished and sweating is likely.

4. Sweating on a cold day is potentially harmful if the runner is dressed warmly and clothing prevents evaporation. The sweat thus tends to remain in the clothing and to

unduly accelerate the rate at which the body is cooled. The effect is comparable to being immersed, and water conducts heat much more rapidly than air. It has been estimated that cold wet clothing conducts heat up to 240 times faster than warm dry clothing.

5. In addition to sweating, the runner will be breathing rapidly, and significant amounts of both heat and moisture will be lost with the expired air. At rest, ten percent of the body's heat and water vapor is lost due to normal respiration; when the individual is working hard, vastly more is lost.

As inspired air enters the body, it is humidified (for the benefit of the alveolar sacs) and warmed. When the air being inspired is cold and dry, more body heat and moisture are required to make it "palatable" to the lungs. As the same air is expired from the body's core, it usually contains even more heat and water vapor, and the effect of heat and water loss experienced through respiration cannot be emphasized strongly enough. *Dehydration is a frequent contributor to the development of hypothermia among outdoor workers and sports and fitness enthusiasts.*

6. Running under warm thermal conditions consumes much energy. Running in the cold consumes even more. As long as energy supplies are adequate and adequate body fluids are maintained, the runner should experience no major difficulties. If, however, the point of fatigue is reached, when readily converted energy sources are exhausted, and the runner continues to run, then hypothermia can quickly result. Thus, in addition to maintaining good physical condition, runners and workers must keep themselves nutritionally fit.

7. Cold air causes an increase in mucous production within the respiratory passages. This is especially common among victims of asthma and persons who have respiratory system problems. When there is a mucous buildup, shortness of breath often develops.

8. Because the heavily exercised (or worked) body is actively engaged in cooling itself, should an accident occur in the cold, it is imperative that immediate steps be taken to

warm the disabled victim. Hypothermia can quickly attack a hot, sweating runner whose energy reserves have been drained by a four- or five-mile run.

One final consideration: recent studies indicate that physically fit people are able to tolerate the cold better than those unaccustomed to exercise or physical labor. Among the reasons for this is the fact that regular exercise has a lasting effect on increased metabolism; that is, metabolism remains more efficient following vigorous exercise.

MOUNTAIN HYPOTHERMIA

Along with polar exploration, mountain climbing, especially at very high altitudes (above 18,000 ft or 5,486 m), is one of the most taxing physical activities men and women engage in. An exercise activity such as jogging, skiing or even marathon running involves exertion for a sustained period of several hours or less, but mountain climbing often involves days, even weeks, of continual stress from physical exertion and exposure. Such prolonged stress exacts a great price from the body and mind.

Many of the concerns discussed in this section are primarily problems existing at higher altitudes. "Mountain sickness," for example, is rare at low altitudes. Climbers, hikers, backpackers, and campers should be particularly attentive, to information herein, as well as to that in the section on work and recreation in the cold.

Mountain heights are notorious for unpredictable weather. Temperatures are nearly always cold and can plummet with hardly any advance warning. Sudden gusts of winds in excess of 40 miles an hour are not uncommon. Blizzards, cold rain, lack of shelter, and the scarcity of fuel for fires make for a hostile, challenging environment. Furthermore, problems of access in the mountains can leave an injured or hypothermic person exposed for many hours or days before rescue.

A great deal has been written about the type of clothing which should be worn in the mountains and there is no need to repeat that advice here. Crucial, however, is the layering of one's clothes, keeping clothing dry, and wearing fabrics, such as wool, which retain warmth. Also, the steel shank boot, which is needed for strong support, is always much colder than the body, and heat loss by conduction from it will occur continually. Heat loss will also occur when the climber touches cold rocks with the hands and body, a condition unavoidable on a climb. As mentioned previously, heat loss by way of respiration, or ventilation, can become a significant factor when one is exercising in the cold because of decreased oxygen pressure at high altitudes which stimulates ventilation and is greater in mountain climbing than in other activities because of decreased oxygen levels at high altitudes.

A study conducted several years ago found that most major mountain ascents which failed did so because of three factors: the climbers did not get enough sleep, meals were uninspiring, and the effects of dehydration. All of these factors contribute to fatigue, and fatigue is hypothermia's doorstep. Once a climber begins to suffer fatigue, resources of fighting hypothermia are easily depleted.

Sleep is difficult when climbing because there is seldom a safe, warm place in which to retreat. Rock, as said, is a good thermal conductor, and the wind, cold and other deleterious elements often literally surround a climber, and the body, even when it is presumably asleep, is always tensed and on the alert. Many mountain climbers believe that if they are in their sleeping bags, they will be able to remain (or become) warm. This is a dangerous assumption since the thermal difference between the body and the environment always results in heat loss. At night, tremendous amounts of heat will be lost primarily through respiration, and through conduction to the cold ground.

Loss of appetite is common on almost all climbs and is related to mountain sickness. Generally the meals and rations which have been planned are nutritious and packed with energy, but, again, they tend to become boring and unappetizing. All the food in the world won't help someone who is unexcited by it and won't eat.

Dehydration is a particular problem since both heat and water vapor are lost in great quantities at high altitude and in cold temperatures. For some reason, people in the cold often are not as aware of their thirst and tend to drink less liquid than their bodies need. Without fluids, metabolism is affected and heat production will not be optimal. Dehydration also contributes to fatigue and increased susceptibility to hypothermia.

At high altitudes the air is less dense and there is less oxygen available. Even at a height of 3,000 feet (914 m), most people experience shortness of breath. The lack of oxygen creates many problems as the body tries to adjust to new "operating conditions," some of which can be overcome; others cannot, but can be "lived with." It is essential for every climber to know what is going on and to act wisely; to do otherwise will jeopardize health and safety.

People can acclimatize to the hostile environments of the high altitudes if they allow themselves enough time. At 18,000 ft, for example, the atmospheric pressure is half of what it is at sea level, but the proportion of oxygen in the air is the same as it was at sea level. The reduction of available oxygen is related to the lower barometric pressure since oxygen uptake by the blood is dependent on the partial *pressure* of oxygen and not on its concentration. As the chemical sensors in the body sense a decrease in oxygen level within the blood, the autonomic nervous system compensates for that shortage by increasing the rate of ventilation. This increased respiratory rate begins at much lower levels for most people.

As the body begins to increase breathing rate, the capillaries in the lungs are more fully perfused with blood, thereby increasing the capacity of the respiratory system to utilize the limited supply of oxygen available. Also, a *gradual* increase in the number of red blood cells in the blood takes place. Since red blood cells carry oxygen from the lungs to all parts of the body, the more red blood cells you have, the better your ability to capture the small amount of oxygen available in the lungs. This reaction is slow at first, but increases over a period of weeks of exposure to reduced oxygen supply.

Also, over a period of time there is an increase in the number of capillaries in skeletal muscle, which helps it work more efficiently with less oxygen. At the same time certain chemicals normally found in the blood increase in concentration to facilitate the release of oxygen to the tissues from the red blood cells.

The rate of these changes varies greatly from person to person, but most are completed in 6–10 days. Unfortunately, many climbers have a limited amount of time to acclimatize and consequently there is a tendency for them to undergo additional stress on their bodies by not allowing these changes to occur gradually.

Once a climber returns to a lower altitude, he will lose acclimatization. The Inca Indians of Peru were aware of this phenomenon and had laws which prohibited those who lived in the lowlands from going to the highlands. The Spanish conquerors found the highlands of Peru so inhospitably cold and life there so arduous that they sent their pregnant women to the lowlands for childbirth, having observed many stillbirths among the Spanish women—but few among the local Indian women. The point, again, is that acclimatization takes time.

The term "mountain sickness" is rather loosely used to describe a series of effects on the body resulting from inadequate acclimatization; that is, the body has not yet fully adjusted to the high altitude environment. The most common symptoms include:

1. headache, dizziness;
2. fatigue;
3. shortness of breath;
4. loss of appetite;
5. nausea, vomiting; and
6. hyperventilation;
7. insomnia

Because these purely physiological stresses are added to those of climbing and fighting the elements, the predisposition to hypothermia is great. Shortness of breath and hyperventilation lead to increased heat loss; loss of appetite has a negative impact on metabolism because adequate energy reserves for heat production are reduced; and vomiting can quickly lead to dehydration and contribute to the overall feeling of fatigue.

Overall, then, the following effects on the body from high altitude can subject the climber to hypothermia and/or frostbite:

Decreased oxygen supplies cut into the efficiency of the body's processes, at least for a time. This can also lead to a loss of concentration, forgetfulness and carelessness, which can, in turn, place the individual in a dangerous situation from which he is incapable of extracting himself.

Lowered oxygen intake leads to decreased metabolic efficiency, diminished work efficiency and heat production.

Heat loss increases with altitude, through the respiratory system, because ventilation is increased; muscle failure of the ventilation system is also common, especially among inexperienced climbers who overextend themselves.

Loss of appetite and dehydration affect energy levels, mental functions, and can quickly lead to the deterioration of other body systems, producing a clearcut reduction in the body's ability to withstand the stress of cold temperatures.

Increased viscosity of the blood can affect respiration, mental functioning and overall organ efficiency, and results in an increased load on the heart.

Each of these disorders accelerates the effects of the other, but all can be handled—if recognized—by returning to a lower altitude and initiating proper rewarming, feeding and medication.

COLD WATER ACCIDENTS, DROWNING AND PERSONAL FLOTATION DEVICES

Swimming and boating accidents probably account for more hypothermia-related deaths than any other single cause. One reason for this is that water conducts heat away from the body 25–30 times faster than air. Another is that muscle rigidity and eventual unconsciousness caused by hypothermia often contribute to death by drowning. Few statistics are available which differentiate water-related death due to hypothermia from those due solely to drowning, but in one northern state water safety officers have estimated that at least one-half of all "drownings" were a result of hypothermia. If the victims had been able to resist hypothermia, drowning might not have occurred.

COLD WATER IMMERSION (IMMERSION HYPOTHERMIA)

The term *cold water* usually refers to water within a temperature range of 32°F and 70°F (0°C–21.1°C). It should be noted, however, that water at any temperature lower than that of the body's core will promote heat loss and thus can contribute to hypothermia. The chart shows the *estimated* survival time for unclothed persons of average weight and body build in water of various temperatures.

Do not assume that just because the water is cold you will die shortly after falling in. Sudden hypothermic death occurs only in water which has become icy slush and when you do not have on any protective gear. The value of wearing protective gear in potentially hypothermic situations should be evident!

When a person suddenly falls (or jumps) into cold water, the progression of events involved in hypothermia begins. This "progression" is discussed in detail in Chapter 4. In addition, several other events occur which affect the rate at which hypothermia (and/or drowning) will develop—assuming no rescue is made.

The Shock Response

Sudden exposure to cold water always involves the respiratory and cardiovascular systems. This response is termed a *respiratory arrest*. The initial gasping response is largely involuntary; that is, you can't help yourself. Once the initial shock is over, most people can refrain from further gasping. However, some find it extremely difficult to control gasping, and they may gasp frantically for several minutes. Such behavior is fatiguing and can easily cause the victim (and others) to panic. Aside from its potential for causing panic, the other real danger associated with gasping is that in rough waters, gasping often leads to the breathing-in of water. Continued gasping alters the chemistry of the blood and may lead to unconsciousness or disorientation. Also cold shock will cause an increase in heart rate and blood pressure and may, in certain cases, cause heart failure.

Pain

The initial experience of cold water immersion is one of pain, and in very cold water, intense pain. Since many people believe that "five minutes in 40°F (4.4°C) water will kill you," that sudden experience of pain often serves to confirm their worst suspicions. Consequently, they give up and wait to die—they usually do, too, not from the water, but from their own lack of will. Survivors are people who are *determined* to survive!

Case reports from survivors of shipwrecks and airplane ditchings, as well as for laboratory experiments, indicate that after a few minutes, such pain subsides or the person at least becomes tolerant of it. The water still feels cold, but that sharp sense of total body pain lessens considerably.

Cold Induced Vasodilatation

The blood vessels serving the skin and the peripheral extremities (especially the fingers) initially constrict, and eventually dilate. The consequence of this response is that heat loss is accelerated. This response is variable and does not always occur in everyone or under all conditions.

Sink or Swim or?

Standing water is able to drain body heat away at a very fast rate. Turbulence, swimming or shivering increase the movement of water across the skin and the rate of heat loss even more. Moving the arms and legs in swimming motions also increases blood flow to those high heat loss areas, thus adding yet another dimension to the problem of rapid body cooling.

Water safety experts recommend that persons in dangerously cold water should *not* swim or move about any more than is absolutely necessary to keep the head and neck out of the water and to stay afloat. The only exceptions are: (1) if you must escape the sucking whirlpools of a sinking vessel, or (2) if a piece of wreckage, a life raft or dry land is *clearly* within reach.

If you do not have a personal flotation device and cannot gain access to a life raft, a piece of wreckage or the shoreline, you must decide what to do to stay afloat. There is some controversy surrounding this issue. Some experts recommend treading water since doing so enables one to keep the head and neck out of the cold water (more or less). The drawback to treading water is that it consumes a lot of energy and it can quickly cause fatigue. Also, because of the body movement required, it accelerates heat loss.

Other experts recommend a technique called "drown-proofing." Basically, the technique involves a gliding through the water face down with relatively little movement of the limbs, with breaths taken when you break the surface of the water. The advantage of this technique is that much less energy is expended and there is not as much movement of the arms and legs. On the other hand, it does require the continued wetting of the head and neck—both areas of dangerous and rapid heat loss.

The head is a critical area of heat loss. The reason is that blood flow to the brain will remain constant even after its flow to other areas has been curtailed. Since approximately 20% of the blood pumped from the heart goes to the brain, it receives a significant amount of the body's heat. Yet the brain has no insulation. It is encased in a bony framework which loses heat rapidly by way of conduction and radiation. Once the head gets cold, it will act as a constant drain on the body. Further, many neural centers which control respiration and circulation are located quite close to the base of the skull. These areas tend to cool rapidly, thus compromising the body's ability to regulate its cardiovascular and respiratory functions. In any hypothermic situation, and especially when on the water, it is essential that the head and neck be protected to ensure long-term survival.

To avoid having to make a choice between the threat of fatigue and exhaustion resulting from treading water and the threat of chilling the head and neck while drown-proofing, *be smart: always wear a personal flotation device!*

Buoyancy

Personal flotation devices will be discussed at a later point: let it simply be said here that they greatly increase buoyancy, conserve energy and help keep the head and neck out of the water. They should be worn by all persons on the water. Whatever inconvenience or discomfort they might cause is more than offset by the extra margin of safety they provide.

In the absence of personal flotation devices, the buoyancy of the body is largely dependent on subcutaneous fat. Very fat persons tend to be quite buoyant and because of the insulating properties of body fat, their core temperature drops much more slowly than does that of very thin people. Women typically have more subcutaneous fat than men of comparable size and weight, so they tend to be slightly more bouyant.

The buoyancy provided by fat is important chiefly because the body will require less energy to keep afloat and thus more energy is available to maintain heat production. The advantage of this extra buoyancy is so great that a fat person may well have three to four times the chance of survival than a thin person. However, fat people may also be less able to generate energy because they are often not physically fit, will not have the biochemical machinery to generate heat efficiently, and will be less able to tolerate the cardiovascular shock.

Clothing

Just as body fat acts as insulation, thereby maintaining favorable core temperatures over a longer time span, clothing serves much the same function, although it is not as effective in this regard as body fat.

Any clothing that a person has on when entering the water should be retained. If one knows that immersion is imminent, it is advisable to don gloves, a watch-cap or other hat, as much warm clothing as can be had, and an exposure suit or windbreaker. All such clothing reduces the movement of water across the skin and thus retards cooling. Certain kinds of shoes (like tennis shoes) and gloves help protect the feet and hands which, as has been mentioned, have a tendency to lose large amounts of heat. Heavy boots (like hiking boots) may inhibit movement of the legs and drag one down.

HELP and Huddle?

Assuming the victim has a personal flotation device, the so-called HELP position *may* be advisable. HELP stands for Heat Escape Lessening Position. To assume this position in the water, one simply draws the knees up to the chest in an approximation of the fetal position. Heat loss is decreased because the person has reduced the amount of body surface exposed to the water, and especially because the groin and chest areas are shielded. These two areas tend to be high

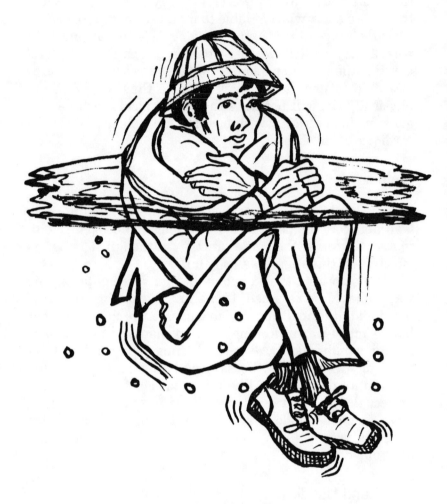

HELP

HELP: The fetus-like Heat Escape Lessening Position, used when wearing a flotation device, can sharply increase cold water survival time.

heat loss areas because they are usually covered with very little fat and major blood vessels are near the surface of the skin.

However, do not try this position in an emergency unless you have tried it with a personal flotation device (identical to the one you have on) in a swimming pool or other "safe" water. The reason for this precaution is that many people roll over backward or forward when assuming this position, thereby chilling the head and neck and, quite possibly, increasing the risk of swallowing water. Since many people are completely unable to assume this position safely, it should be tested in the safety of a swimming pool before it's needed in an emergency.

As an alternative to the HELP position, heat loss can be reduced slightly by crossing the legs at the ankles and bringing the thighs together. It is also advisable to keep the arms crossed, close against the chest.

The so-called *huddle* position is recommended for groups of three or more people; it refers to the interlocking of arms (or wrapping them around each other) to keep bodies close together. The somewhat circular formation which results will reduce the circulation of water across the chests of the participants. Some believe the water in the center will be warmed by the bodies. The main advantages of this procedure are that it keeps the members of the party together and it provides the opportunity for psychological support, an important element in survival.

When rescuing a victim found floating in cold water, one should determine if the person (a) is dead, (b) is in deep hypothermia as a result of immersion, or (c) is suffering from *both* hypothermia and asphyxia. (This latter condition is termed submersion hypothermia.)

Differentiating between these conditions is critical since it will determine the course of action. One rule of thumb is that if the victim is wearing a life jacket and the waters are not too rough, he is probably suffering from immersion hypothermia.

Although the major points to be considered in rescue and rewarming are covered in Chapter 8, two major issues

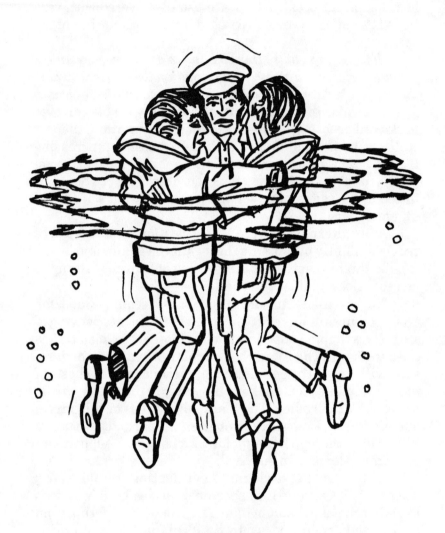

HUDDLE

Huddle: This position is recommended for three or more people. In addition to reducing heat loss, it helps keep them from becoming separated.

associated with immersion hypothermia deserve to be mentioned here.

The first of these matters deals with the effect of water pressure on the body (hydrostatic squeeze). Rescuers of immersion hypothermia victims should be aware of the fact that such victims often faint after being pulled from the water. The reason for this is that so long as the person's body was in the water, water compressed the superficial blood vessels in much the same way that "support hose" does. Once that support is withdrawn, there is a tendency for the blood to "rush" from the brain and core into the peripheral areas, causing a temporary fainting. There is also a sudden reduction in the amount of blood ejected from the heart, causing the victim to pass out; if these complications are severe enough, they may cause cardiac arrhythmias and death. Always place an immersion hypothermia victim in a horizontal position with the head slightly lower than the legs.

The second matter deals with "rewarming collapse." Except when immersion hypothermia victims are rewarmed slowly and spontaneously, there is danger of fainting and cardiac arrhythmias and death. These developments arise due to the rapid dilation of blood vessels in the peripheral areas. Furthermore, rapid warming of the skin will cause the body to release the neural controls which have been maintaining systemic blood pressure. This action can also cause a variety of cardiovascular problems.

When an immersion hypothermia victim is *conscious, alert,* and *shivering,* warm baths or showers may be permitted *under close supervision.*

COLD WATER SUBMERSION

This section might be more aptly referred to as "hypothermic considerations in cold water drowning." When a person is submerged in cold water (i.e., all the way under), there are two threats to survival: hypothermia and oxygen deprivation (anoxia).

THE DIVE REFLEX

Neural reflexes occur in response to a very specific stimulus over which the conscious mind has very little control. The dive reflex is a response triggered by the sudden contact of very cold water with the face, such as might occur when diving or falling into a cold lake. There is some evidence to indicate that the sudden inhalation of very cold air may trigger a similar response via receptors in the lungs. In humans, this stimulus causes three simultaneous reactions within the body: (1) a significant decrease in heart rate; (2) a vasoconstriction of the blood vessels in the periphery; and (3) an increase in blood pressure, apparently as a result of vasoconstriction.

These actions serve to help protect the brain from anoxia, or severe oxygen deprivation. Theoretically, this reflex action shunts blood from the peripheral areas to the trunk of the body where it can serve the vital organs. Thus, even though the person may not be breathing, an adequate supply of oxygenated blood is available to maintain critical life support functions.

A pronounced cold stimulus to the face from either water or air can sometimes slow the heart to the degree that a heart attack will occur! Thus the dive reflex isn't always a friend.

While this reflex is usually a survival aid, its value as such is greatly augmented by the entire body's response to cold water immersion or submersion. It will be recalled that in cold water conductive heat loss is quite rapid. This loss triggers the same three initial reactions that the dive reflex does, albeit somewhat more slowly. In terms of survival, the overall cooling effect of the water is probably more important than the dive reflex is in the shunting of blood from the periphery to the core.

Although the precise mechanism is not fully understood, a related action, which occurs when the face and head are suddenly submerged in cold water, is a slowing down of the brain and other organ systems. This *rapid* cooling (and the subsequent decrease in oxygen requirements) happens

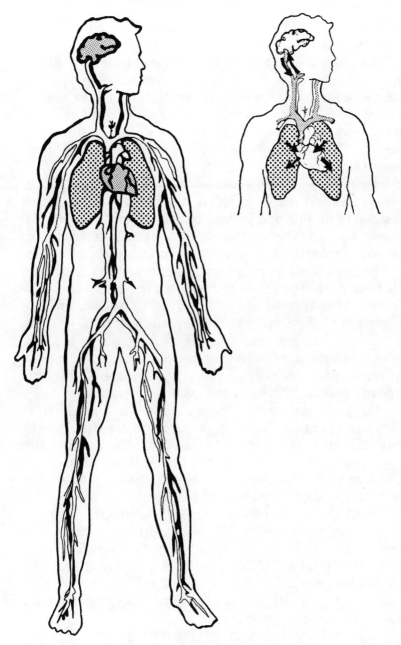

In the dive reflex, circulation of the blood to the limbs is shunted to the lungs, heart, and brain, thereby prolonging function of the vital organs. Also critically important, as the heart rate drops the blood pressure rises.

much faster in cold water submersion than it does in most other exposure situations.

The combined effects of these reflex actions have been known to sustain children who have been submerged in very cold water for nearly an hour. Resuscitation and revival is a difficult undertaking for even the most skilled of physicians, and such victims often suffer pulmonary complications and, occasionally, brain damage (especially at the warmer temperatures).

Two related observations may be of interest. First, responsiveness to the dive reflex appears to be more pronounced in infants and young children than it is in adults. Second, the reflex seems to occur faster and to last longer if the person is partially exhaling when his face hits the water.

Because the dive reflex and other associated hypothermic responses so completely shut down the body, it is possible for a person to be fully submerged in cold water for a longer time before dying than in warm water.

True drowning is caused when a person is actually suffocated by water. Drowning causes many complications within the body, including pulmonary edema, but the cause of death is usually anoxia, or oxygen deprivation.

Oxygen deprivation occurs chiefly when a person is submerged because the lungs, sooner or later, fill up with water. The presence of water in the lungs makes it virtually impossible for oxygen to combine with the blood. (Fish can do it; people can't!) In order for the blood to be oxygenated, the water must be removed from the lungs.

Since the brain is more sensitive to oxygen deprivation than any other organ, it will begin to malfunction fairly soon—within three to four minutes at air temperatures in the 80–90°F (26.6–32.2°C) range. Here we can see the importance of the dive reflex, for if it successfully shunts blood to meet the brain's oxygen requirements, the victim stands a much better chance of survival.

Unless doing so would endanger your own life, every effort should be made to revive any cold water submersion victim. When in doubt, try anyway. Of all possible victims, little children stand the best chance of surviving long-term cold water submersion. There are three reasons for this. First, as stated, the dive reflex is stronger in small children than in anyone else. Second, children cool off faster than adults. The result of this is that their metabolic and neural functions "shut down" sooner. Finally, for reasons which are not fully understood, infants and young children are better able to withstand prolonged periods of anoxia.

Rescue and resuscitation of the cold water *submersion* victim are tricky. One must first remove the water in the lungs so that blood can be oxygenated; only then is rewarming of the victim recommended. If rewarming occurs before the blood is oxygenated and before respiration can take place, the warmed brain will require more oxygen than it has access to and will suffer anoxia. Anoxia often leads to brain damage or death. The procedures to follow, then, should be the same as those used for CPR (Cardiopulmonary Resuscitation):

1. clear the airways of any obstruction;
2. perform artificial ventilation;
3. perform external chest compression; and
4. rewarm the victim.

A word of caution: even though a submerged person is rescued and successfully revived, he or she should be watched closely and transported to a medical facility as soon as possible. The term *near drowning* is used to refer to the many persons who die following an apparently successful resuscitation and revival. Near-drowning deaths occur within 24 hours of rescue and are fairly common.

THE PERSONAL FLOTATION DEVICES (PFDs) AND THERMAL PROTECTION IN THE WATER

As has been noted, thermal conductivity of water is quite high. Thermal protection in cold water is accordingly a grave concern for those persons whose recreational or occupational pursuits place them on the water. Industrial and military personnel typically have somewhat more knowledge about personal flotation devices than the average citizen who is a weekend boater, but many organizations fail to educate their employees properly, to provide adequate equipment and to insist that safety precautions be followed. Often only after a fatality has occurred do people remember the old adage: an ounce of prevention is worth a pound of cure!

It is extremely important to realize that the primary purpose of personal flotation devices is to assist in keeping a person afloat by providing extra buoyancy. Some PFDs also provide nominal thermal protection, but that is not their primary purpose.

The Coast Guard has approved five types of PFD. Their characteristics are described below.

Type I is designed to rotate a person's body from a face down (in the water) position to a vertical or slightly backward, upright position. This rotation process should occur within 2–3 seconds. These PFDs are very bulky and are found on ocean-going vessels for emergency use only.

Type II devices are typically used in institutional settings and for "adapted aquatic" programs for handicapped persons. These are the familar orange yoke PFDs. They may rotate the wearer, but the turning action is not as strong or as rapid as in Type I.

Type III are the most common PFDs in use. The vests or flotation jackets come in many colors. They allow the wearer to position himself in an upright posture, but the device itself may not rotate the body. Once positioned, the wearer should be able to remain vertical or at a slightly backward slant. These PFDs are the least bulky and usually the most comfortable when worn out of the water.

Type IV are designed to be thrown to a person in the water. An example is the floatable seat cushion often found on boats. They provide buoyancy, but have no particular positioning characteristics since they are usually not worn.

Type V PFDs are approved by the Coast Guard and are designed for specialty uses such as speed-boat racers, oil rig workers, etc., and are sometimes specially constructed for hypothermia protection.

Some incidental hypothermia protection is provided by a PFD to the extent that it allows the person to remain afloat without exertion. The more the floater splashes around, the greater the heat loss. Also, by keeping the face and neck out of the water, heat loss from those vulnerable areas is reduced.

An important precaution which should be taken is to try out the actual personal flotation device you would use should an emergency occur. The reason for this admonition is that various PFDs behave differently with different people, because each person's buoyancy characteristics are different.

The major determinant of personal buoyancy is body fat. Fat is lighter than water; it floats. Muscle mass and bone are heavier than water; they tend to sink. The position in which you float, independent of PFD, is a function of the way muscle and fat are distributed in your body. Persons who have large fat deposits around the hips and buttocks will have difficulty maintaining an upright position because that portion of their anatomy will have a natural tendency to rise to the surface; as a consequence, their head and shoulders will be forced down into the water.

Because your particular body build will behave in a unique way with each personal flotation device, it is especially important that a trial immersion be conducted, just to be certain that your head and neck will be supported out of the water. Trying out such devices with children and handicapped persons is mandatory. Based on their size and body weight, most children have a disproportionately heavy head and not all PFDs will support them in the desired position. Also, since with each phase of growth the child's distribution of muscle and fat changes, frequent tests of the PFD are recommended.

With the physically handicapped, special problems arise. Under normal conditions, when a person falls into cold

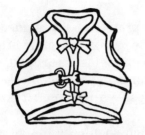

LIFE PRESERVER
(Jacket Type)

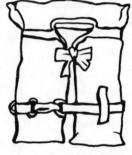

BUOYANT VEST

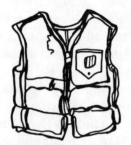

**SPECIAL PURPOSE
BUOYANT DEVICE**

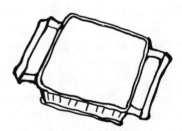

BUOYANT CUSHION

Typical approved flotation devices used for protection under various conditions.

water, a number of reflexes occur. All, such as muscle tensing, are interrelated and coordinated. However, many physically handicapped persons experience poor coordination or an exaggeration of these reflexes. Thus, a handicapped person's muscles might tense up to the point that the legs would be drawn up tightly to the chest. This alters the distribution of fat and muscle, and buoyancy is affected. Many PFDs will not respond safely to a buoyancy shift of this type. Furthermore, many devices (especially Type III) require a certain amount of physical movement if the person is to remain fully upright. Some handicapped persons may not be able to provide this stabilizing movement. Nor can a normal person, if unconscious.

In general, PFDs commonly available do not provide protection against hypothermia, nor do they address the specific disabilities and buoyancy problems of physically handicapped people or other persons with neuromuscular difficulties of various types.

There are two types of survival suits which do provide thermal protection in cold water. These suits come in whole and half-body varieties, and the whole body suits are available as either wet or dry suits.

The whole body dry suit is designed so that no water will enter the suit and a layer of air between the fabric and the body adds to the insulating quality of the suit's construction material. While the types of fabrics used in these suits vary considerably, they are all designed to give extended protection in cold water. A typical dry suit should protect an individual for six hours in water at 32°F; protection is defined as preventing more than a 3.6°F (2°C) drop in core temperature. The chief disadvantage of these suits is that they must be worn properly if they are to give protection. In emergency situations, people often do not have time to put the garments on in the recommended fashion.

Whole body wet suits allow a little water next to the body. Theoretically, the body warms this film of water and the warm water then acts as an insulating barrier. Ideally, these suits prevent core temperature drops of more than 3.6°F (2°C) for three hours in 50°F (10°C) water. The major problem with these suits is that they are very hot and clumsy when worn on a day-to-day basis and many industrial workers simply won't wear them.

By way of compromise, the half-body wet suit was developed. These suits cover the shoulders and trunk of the body; they have a flap of material which covers the hips and buttocks and comes around in front between the legs to cover the groin region. These suits offer a fairly high degree of protection, and are lighter and somewhat more comfortable to wear. Again, they offer protection for three hours in 50°F (10°C) water.

Ideally, the suits are donned before the person enters the water. Some wet suits are purportedly designed to be put on in the water, but doing so is often very difficult in choppy seas.

SCUBA DIVING

Scuba diving is not only one of the world's fastest growing recreational activities, it and deep-water diving are being used for an ever-broadening range of commercial and industrial purposes. Because water is so efficient as a thermal conductor, hypothermia is a major problem for both recreational and professional divers. The chilling effects of both fresh and salt water dives are such that wet suits are required for virtually all dives except those in shallow tropical waters. In addition to wet suits, a variety of other diving suits and diving bells are used to provide divers with the protection they need at greater depths or in particularly cold waters.

Shallow water divers, as well as those who engage in deep diving, also face the problem of heat loss. Many inland lakes are quite cold, even at depths of 15–35 feet (4.6–10.7 m), and the increasing popularity of ice-diving subjects the diver to severe temperatures. Numbness and all of the other symptoms of hypothermia can take over the body very quickly. Obviously, hypothermic insult while underwater is an immediate health hazard. Another problem associated with diving and the cold is nausea induced by cold water entering a broken eardrum.

Wet suits are thought to protect most divers when the suits are properly worn, but even a properly fitted suit cannot completely prevent heat loss. When a diver's wet suit is not fitted properly, too much cold water will stream through, accelerating heat loss; this effect can also be created by a cut or tear in the fabric of the suit. Divers should also note (if they haven't found out the hard way) that wet suits provide good protection only down to 60 feet (18.2 m) since beyond that point increased pressure will decrease the insulation value of the neoprene foam used in the suits. As the foam's air pockets are compressed, heat loss is accelerated by conduction and convection.

Most divers seem to prefer the wet suit because it is easier to put on and the shock of a rip or tear is not so sudden. Dry suits can be worn over thermal underwear, but the diver must compensate for the added buoyancy.

In recent years, there has been an increased use of warm humidified air by divers. Such air obviously warms the core, but it induces peripheral vasodilatation in many people. This vasodilatation can easily mislead the central nervous system into believing that the body is warmer than it actually is. Should this happen, the body will not mount its normal defenses against hypothermia and the diver can easily reach a critical point before becoming aware of the danger. While it is true that the risks of hypothermia are especially great at lower levels, critical heat loss can occur even in warm, shallow waters.

HYPOTHERMIA AND THE ELDERLY

Hypothermia is a continuing and all-pervasive threat to the elderly. More than any other single group of people, the aged are confronted with the problem of keeping warm on an almost daily basis. They are most vulnerable to temperature changes and least able to protect themselves. Unfortunately, scientists are only beginning to understand the many complications that the aged experience with thermoregulation, and public policy lags far behind what knowledge we do have. The frequent personal neglect which many older people experience makes them all the more vulnerable, both physically and psychologically. A great deal of research and a social shouldering of responsibility needs to take place to meet the needs of the elderly with respect to hypothermia.

Hypothermia poses a great threat to the elderly because the aging process decreases the effectiveness of many of the body's thermal protective mechanisms; also, the development of health problems common to old age further complicate the older person's ability to maintain adequate body warmth.

No single profile adequately defines the health status of the elderly; the changes which occur naturally do so at different rates for each individual, and any specific health problem which may arise in one person will not necessarily appear in the next. The topics discussed below are most frequently encountered with the elderly. The extent to which any one (or more) of these factors will affect people varies widely across the country. It should be emphasized that old age does not necessarily "cause" any specific disease or disorder. The first four problems listed below, for example, can develop without any overt sign of illness.

Decreased Sensory Perception and Altered Neural Function

As the aging process continues, there appears to be a gradual but progressive decrease in the body's ability to detect changes in its sensory input. Among the elderly, it often appears that the thermoreceptors either do not detect cold as effectively as they once did, or if they do, that an inappropriate message is reaching the brain. In an impaired detection system, all reflexes and responses which would normally occur in reaction to the cold will be delayed or nonexistent.

Decreased Muscle Mass and Decreased Shivering

Many elderly people have a significant decrease in their muscle mass, and therefore appear to be skinny. This reduction in muscle mass is not necessarily disabling, but it does adversely affect the individual's ability to shiver. Among many older people, the neuromuscular control network for shivering also is not as effective and shivering will sometimes not occur even though the person might feel quite cold.

"Chronic" Inactivity

Many older people are highly inactive. Disease, boredom and neglect often contribute to chronic inactivity. Persons confined to the bed or to a wheelchair because of broken bones, strokes, paralysis, arthritis or various other crippling disabilities are particularly prone to hypothermia because of their inactivity. Some victims of Parkinson's disease are also often relatively inactive, but their plight is further complicated by their predisposition to excessive sweating and flushing of the skin.

Decreased Metabolic Rate

For a variety of reasons, some of which are still not understood, many elderly people have a decreased metabolic rate. This lower level of metabolic activity may occur rather suddenly, or it can develop gradually. In either case, once the basal metabolic rate is altered so that the constant level of warmth being produced is lowered, then the person is much more susceptible to bodily insult from the cold.

Malnutrition

Starvation and malnutrition lead quickly to other disorders and conditions which weaken the victim's resistance. Depending on the specific way that starvation and malnutrition manifest themselves in a given individual, there could be cardiovascular, respiratory, or nervous system involvement. To the extent that any one of these systems is compromised, so too will the victim be in danger of hypothermia.

Starvation and malnutrition are a concern in the elderly since so many of them attempt to live on inadequate or marginal diets. Also, many older people have gastrointestinal problems or other diseases, such as severe anemia, which can indirectly affect their nutritional status, thus predisposing them to hypothermia.

Strokes

The term *stroke* refers to any one of a variety of cerebrovascular accidents which destroy brain tissue. Some people recover the affected functions; more often, the damage is permanent. As people get older, there is an increased susceptibility to strokes, many of which are so minor as to escape detection, but they can still lead to the loss of some brain function. If a person experiences one or more strokes in the areas of the brain which monitor or control thermoregulation, the ability to respond to cold will be affected. Such strokes can also affect the ability to detect cold, as well as to take an appropriate defensive or protective action.

Medication

The elderly are commonly on medications for the treatment of various disorders. Of these medications, some compromise neuronal cell functioning. Others alter blood flow or metabolic rate. In particular, medications used for high blood pressure control, sleep production, tranquilization and mood elevation have the potential for inducing hypothermia. It can also be induced in younger people by the same drugs, but the nervous systems of older persons are apparently somewhat more susceptible to their impact.

Accidents

Older people often have difficulty maintaining their balance and footing, particularly during the winter months when steps, sidewalks and walkways are icy or snow-covered. Because their bones are more likely to fracture, and because it is often a problem for them to regain an upright position once they have fallen, the elderly are easily rendered helpless by a fall. Quite apart from any injury which might occur during a fall, the fact that the person is left lying helpless on the floor or ground is sufficient to bring on hypothermia.

A related threat stems from the fact that the elderly are often the victims of assault, vandalism and other crimes that leave them disabled or injured. For these reasons, family or group living arrangements are highly recommended; if the elderly person lives alone, someone should check in with him or her at least once each day.

Vascular Difficulties

Arteriosclerosis and a variety of other disorders of the blood vessels can lead to a decreased ability for vasoconstriction or vasodilatation. Since these processes are critical to the distribution of warm blood throughout the body, such problems can severely interfere with thermoregulation.

Mental Health and Central Nervous System Problems

Among the elderly, there is often (but by no means always) a mild to severe deterioration of centrally mediated neuromuscular functions. At times these behavioral and functional problems are the result of strokes or other identifiable disorders; at others the aging process itself appears to take its toll on the brain. In either event, the body does not respond as quickly to external stimuli as it once did, nor in as effective a manner as might be desired.

It is also thought that old people do not have the same temperature cycle that they had when they were young. They thus may feel cool during the day and warmer at night.

Certain mental disorders found among the elderly, such as depression, senility and disorientation, are often related to a more widespread central nervous system involvement, and thermoregulatory processes may be compromised as well.

Clothing and Shelter

Although the problem of inadequate clothing and shelter is much more pronounced in the northern latitudes, elderly persons everywhere wear garments that for them no longer have the warmth-retention benefits they once provided. The homes and apartments of older persons are often allowed to fall into disrepair, and even such a seemingly insignificant matter as a poorly caulked window can cause hypothermia. (Chapter 9 contains suggestions for preventing hypothermia among the elderly.)

HYPOTHERMIA IN INFANTS AND SMALL CHILDREN

Hypothermia is a particular problem for young children and infants. For the newborn, there are any number of factors working against heat conservation. As an example, the infant has a relatively large surface area for its body weight, a low level of subcutaneous fat, a relatively thin skin and a high concentration of body fluid (predominately water) in the skin. The infant's skin also has a higher-than-average permeability, so it is especially predisposed to heat loss. Perhaps the major disadvantage which infants suffer is the fact that shivering typically occurs as a much later development in hypothermia than it does in adults. Thus, if an infant is shivering, the chances are the core temperature has already dropped several degrees. There is also evidence to indicate that shivering in infants may not produce heat to the degree that it does in adults, possible due to immaturity of the skeletal muscle.

Premature infants and those unusually light in weight when born often have immature nervous systems and their metabolic processes may not be operating efficiently. Even young children may have a somewhat delayed shivering reaction, and if they are not well-nourished, they tend to fatigue quickly. Infants and young children are also at a particular disadvantage in that they can seldom take any protective action; that is, they cannot seek shelter, put on extra clothing or build a fire. *At least* until the age of four or five, most are completely dependent on adults for protection.

One such example happened recently when a couple went cross-country skiing with their one-year-old son. The child was wearing winter clothing and was riding in a pack carried on the father's back. The air temperature was 20°F (−6.6°C) and there was very little wind. The parents were exercising so much that they were sweating and quite warm. Because they were warm, they assumed the child was too. Unfortunately, he wasn't. The insulation of the father's clothing and the pack kept the child insulated from the adult's body heat. Because the child was not exercising or even moving, he became hypothermic and died.

Infant mortality from hypothermia is common, but even when intervention occurs and the child recovers, long-term effects can result. For the rest of a child's life, growth, blood sugar and endocrine problems may exist because of hypothermia in early childhood. Infants and very young children do have one advantage over adults, in that they are capable of an activity known as nonshivering thermogenesis.

Shivering in adults, it will be recalled, is a powerful heat producing activity which often ward off the development of hypothermia. Nonshivering thermogenesis is another heat-producing phenomenon that relies on certain, apparently specialized, body cells for heat production. These cells are called *brown fat cells*. There is some evidence that skeletal muscle cells may also act to generate heat without shivering, but scientists have a far from complete under-standing of either of these two types of cells.

The extent to which brown fat cells can generate heat varies greatly among mammals. Small species are able to generate proportionately more heat in this manner than large ones, hibernating species more than nonhibernating ones, and newborn animals more than adult animals. Animals which have lived in cold temperatures for long periods of time will utilize such cells more than one newly arrived in a cold climate.

In humans brown fat tissue is found primarily on the upper chest, the armpit region, and the upper back between the shoulder blades. Little is known about the way these cells work. Their unique function appears to be activated by the hormone norepinephrine, which causes the brown fat cells to drastically increase their rate of combustion of food-stuffs and a consequent increase in heat production and dissipation. As these fat cells metabolize, their heat is picked up by the blood which is moving though the cells and carried to the rest of the body. Because this mechanism for heat production requires a good supply of norepinephrine, glucose and oxygen, the premature infant, or one that is small and feeble, or one that has difficulty in breathing, will be placed at a distinct disadvantage. Under cold stress an infant's upper back will typically be one to one-and-a half degrees warmer than the lower back, and there is some evidence that by using its brown fat cells, the infant is able to triple its heat production.

Because of this ability to generate heat without shivering—by using brown fat cells *and* quite possibly its skeletal muscle cells—an infant is able to delay the shiver-ing response. For this reason, as noted, the infant who is shivering has probably already exhausted much of its metabolic resources in warding off the cold.

RACIAL DIFFERENCES

Relatively little research has been done which sys-tematically sorts out racial differences in the body's response to the cold. There are many reasons for our lack of knowledge in this regard, not the least of which is the fact that the term *racial* has little meaning to the biologist. Over the hundreds of thousands of years that humans have been on earth, there has been such an extensive mixing of the world-wide gene pool that "pure" races no longer exist, if in fact they ever did. Nonetheless, "physical" anthropologists and physiologists have compiled some evidence of genetic links to certain types of cold adaptation in humans.

For example, scientists have found that when the whole body is cooled, Euroamericans show a fairly predictable metabolic rate increase. American blacks show the same type of increase, although the response is slower and the body surface seems to undergo greater cooling. Eskimos, on the other hand, show a much more rapid increase in metabolic rate, and their skin temperatures will be more highly elevated. Eskimos also seem to exhibit a more rapid and extensive warming of the fingers and toes, as well as the hands and feet. Having fingers and hands which remain warm, even though they may be immersed in icy water, places the Eskimo in a vulnerable position with respect to heat loss. However, that risk is apparently outweighed by the extra survival value of being able to maintain manual dexterity.

The same type of relationship exists with regard to laboratory studies of hand-rewarmings when the hand is immersed in cold water. Eskimos and North Asian stock peoples (including western hemisphere Indians) typically show less cooling effect and a more rapid rewarming. Also, Eskimos have a basal metabolic rate 20–40% higher than European-stock peoples.

Studies within the American military have found that in Alaska and Korea, black soldiers developed frostbite and other cold injuries more frequently and more rapidly than whites. However, the studies did not demonstrate that genetic factors were responsible for these differences. Beyond these rather broad observations, little can be said relative to genetic adaptations to the cold.

A related topic, that of acclimatization, refers to the

adjustment individuals make to environmental conditions after frequent and prolonged exposure. The scientific literature from the fields of biology, physical anthropology and related disciplines shows that just about everyone is able to adapt to a wide variety of climatic conditions. Such difficulties as are experienced tend to be related to an individual's physiology rather than to any special genetic characteristic.

In addition to acclimatization, which is a biological response to external conditions, humans are also blessed with *cultural adaptation*. This term implies that men and women everywhere learn from each other and exchange information from generation to generation. The adoption of Eskimo "ways," including diet, clothing and transportation, greatly facilitated Peary's strike for the North Pole. Edmund Hillary, the great mountain climber, once commented that Roald Amundsen's reliance on Eskimo-style equipment and travel lore was the key to his speed and efficiency in his race to the South Pole. Robert Scott's use of shetland ponies and motor sledges illustrates that we *don't always learn* from others; Scott reached the pole a month after Amundsen had been there, and died from hypothermia and starvation on his return trip.

The ability to learn from and to build on the wisdom of others plays a far greater role in coping with the cold than does genetics, "race," or physiological adaptation.

CHAPTER 7

Frostbite

Frostbite is the term used to refer to injuries that include actual freezing of deep bodily tissues. Such injuries most commonly affect the peripheral extremities: feet and toes, hands and fingers, nose, ears, cheeks and chin. Among wintertime joggers, frostbite has also been known to affect the breasts and nipples as well as the penis.

While frostbite commonly occurs when the victim is exposed to very cold, dry temperatures, the combined impact of wind and low temperatures (wind-chill effect) can cause it even when the thermometer registers well above freezing. Also, it can, and often does, occur independent of hypothermia. A drop in central body temperature is not a precondition, although developing hypothermia does not necessarily mean the victim will also incur frostbite. The two afflictions are often associated, however, and hypothermia is frequently a contributing factor in its development. This is because the shunting of blood away from the extremities (including such rapid heat-loss areas as the ears and cheeks) allows those body parts to cool very quickly, sometimes to the point of freezing.

Frostbite is a special problem at high altitudes chiefly because heat loss there is much more pronounced. Since less oxygen is being inhaled, there is also less for the blood to deliver to individual cells. Certain high-priority organs (like the heart and brain) receive the lion's share, while cells in the fingers and ears, for example, receive far less. As a consequence, cellular metabolism is reduced disproportionately in the extremities. In addition to the shunting of warm blood, cells are producing less heat on their own. No wonder, then, that they cool so rapidly. However, frostbite is not just a high-altitude mountaineer's disorder. It readily attacks unsuspecting or unprepared victims at all altitudes, and it has brought many an army, both ancient and modern, to a complete standstill.

Two disorders somewhat similar to frostbite, trenchfoot and immersion foot, are especially common among infantry soldiers. These ailments involve tissue damage resulting from prolonged exposure to "frigid" (32–50°F or 0–10°C) water or cold, wet clothing. Very serious injuries can result both from these conditions and the subsequent difficulties they cause for blood vessels, circulation and cellular metabolism.

Frostnip is a term sometimes used when just the skin and the immediately adjacent tissue are frozen. It can develop quite rapidly in cold, windy conditions and is very much like freeze-drying the skin. The surface of the affected area is fairly firm to the touch, but below the surface, the tissue is still vital and resilient. Among Caucasians, the affected skin has a white, waxy sheen to it. Rarely is there any tissue damage, unless the tissue has been rubbed. The standard remedy is rewarming by holding the affected part in direct contact with a warm portion of one's own or a companion's body—placing a warm hand against a frost-nipped cheek, for example. Ice and snow should *never* be applied!

In contrast to frostnip, frostbite always involves tissue damage, and the freezing extends much deeper, often to the bone. In severe cases, not only are dermal and epidermal skin tissues destroyed, but severe injury can be found in the blood vessels, nerves, muscles and even the bones. Full recovery is often possible if rewarming and post-warming care are properly managed. Surgical amputations as well as skin grafting are used far less frequently now than they were in previous decades, but they must still be employed as a last resort in treating some cases.

As with frostnip, the surface of the skin becomes waxy, or even translucent. Unlike frostnip, the underlying tissue becomes hardened, literally taking on the texture of partially thawed meat, which it is. Once thawing occurs, gross discoloration and a variety of other symptoms emerge.

The freezing process typical of frostbite occurs as follows:

Under normal conditions, heat from metabolic functions keeps the skin (which *can* freeze at – .5°C or just under 32°F) soft, pliable and warm. However, when a hand or foot, for example, is exposed to severe cold, heat loss is very rapid because these extremities have so much surface area. Once triggered by thermal receptors, the sympathetic nervous system causes the blood vessels serving the arteries in the extremity to vasoconstrict, thus shunting warm blood away from the "high heat loss zone." At the same time, progressive heat loss and the freezing of superficial tissue causes the blood serving those tissues to become highly viscous. This sludge-like blood literally plugs up the capillaries serving the extremity.

Depending on the severity and duration of the cold, the nervous system may allow some, very little, or no blood to reach the cells in the affected extremity. With their supply of nutrients and oxygen so greatly diminished, the cells are highly vulnerable to external forces—such as the cold (or the abrasiveness of rubbing!).

Extreme cold penetrates the skin and causes ice crystals to form *between* the cells which comprise the tissues. Each such cell is bathed in a solution of intercellular fluid, and it is from this fluid that the first ice crystals form. In turn, the development of ice crystals upsets the chemical and physical processes which help the cell membranes to maintain their structural integrity, sometimes to the point of causing the cell walls literally to burst! As these pressures and the cellular membranes are disrupted, the internal cellular machinery breaks down, sometimes irreparably.

Medical experts have yet to reach a consensus on a classification for frostbite, mainly because the appearance of the affected area varies little from victim to victim; only after rewarming has taken place can the extent of the deep tissue damage be determined. Even then, it may be weeks before an accurate assessment of the damage can be made. For practical purposes, we can classify frostbite as either mild or serious, although within the "serious" category there are several levels of severity.

Mild frostbite leaves the skin swollen and with some blistering. This swelling may last several hours, but within a reasonably short time, swelling and blisters will subside. The skin will remain red and tender for some time.

Within all levels of more serious frostbite, the skin will also be blistered. Such blisters will quite often be large, sometimes reaching the size of large plums or even peaches. *Under no circumstances should they be broken or incised; they contain vital fluids which will eventually be reabsorbed and will facilitate the regeneration of healthy tissue.*

At the first level of severity, the victim will be left with a lack of sensation and temporary muscular paralysis. Both nerve and muscle tissue have been damaged, and the loss of feeling and mobility may last for several weeks.

At the next level, muscle tissue will actually have been destroyed. The skin will eventually heal and appear normal, but the muscle tissue under the skin will never completely recover. Muscle tissue which has been destroyed will, over time, be replaced by fibrous connective tissue. The muscles themselves will lose much of their previous functional capability, the extent being dependent on the degree of injury.

At the third level of severity, the skin is badly damaged, as is much of the underlying muscle tissue. As with the other levels of serious frostbite, there will be extensive blistering initially. Over time, much of skin, and finger or toe nails, will slough off. As this dead tissue is separated from the body, the victim will be left with a very thin, shiny red "skin" which is actually the first or "regerminative" layer of the skin. This skin will be extremely sensitive to both touch and temperature, and it will be highly reactive to cold stimuli.

Months will be required for the body to grow a new skin tissue to cover the affective area.

At the worst level, there is extensive destruction of the skin, muscle, nerves and blood vessels. In many cases, even the bones will have been affected. As the victim thaws, affected body parts will turn a dusky blue–gray and will remain swollen and paralyzed. There will be no sensation. As time passes, the affected parts will turn almost coal black; this is the point at which mummification sets in. Mummification refers to a state of dry gangrene; the cells are actually dead and putrefying. The affected parts no longer have any functional relationship with the body and, as dead tissue, should be amputated.

In previous decades frostbite victims were often isolated from other hospital patients because of their agonized cries and moans, their often grotesque appearance, and the odor of the decaying body parts. Recent advances in treatment have made isolation no longer necessary, but frostbite is still a highly discomforting affliction.

TREATMENT

Early response to frostnip and frostbite can easily prevent much more serious problems. In outdoor situations where frostbite may be a problem, a system of buddy-checks is recommended whereby people examine each others' faces frequently for signs of waxiness and blanching. At the first indication of such symptoms, stop and provide surface to surface contact between warm skin and the affected area. (Remember, no rubbing!) Tell-tale signs in one person are an indication that frostbite may well be on its way for all.

Another early warning sign is the sudden numbing of what were previously just cold extremities. Whenever numbness sets in, immediate rewarming is imperative. It is especially important if socks, gloves or other articles of clothing have become moistened by sweat, melted snow or water. Any wet garment must be removed, the skin dried and warmed, and fresh, dry clothing should be put on.

Once frostbite has actually set in, the affected areas

should not be rewarmed until the victim is completely *out of danger of further exposure to the cold.* Rewarming followed by refreezing causes extensive damage, far more than would have occurred if the affected part were simply left in its frostbitten state. It may be somewhat uncomfortable for the victim to walk on frostbitten feet, but no harm will be done. There are many instances in which mountain climbers have descended several thousand feet with severe frostbite and have recovered fully. There are, on the other hand, very few, if any, cases in which warmed and refrozen extremities have survived functionally intact.

When the feet are involved, once rewarming has begun gross blistering will develop and the victim will be unable to put on shoes or to walk. Transportation by stretcher will be required. Again, rewarming should be initiated only after safety has been reached and the victim is in a location from which medical evacuation will be likely.

When dealing with frostbite in the field, one must also be certain to first treat the victim for hypothermia, if it exists. Hypothermia is a more serious health threat than frostbite, and the control mechanisms which govern body response to lowered core temperatures will dominate those that govern circulation to the extremities. So, it is more important to treat hypothermia first, and thereby ensure survival of basic life support mechanisms, than it is to treat a frostbitten hand or foot.

The method of treating frostbite that is currently most highly recommended is *rapid rewarming.* This approach consistently results in preservation of a greater amount of tissue and a higher degree of function than with any other rewarming procedure. Rapid rewarming is accomplished by immersing the affected part in water maintained at a temperature of 108–112°F (42–44°C). Do not allow the foot or hand to rest on the bottom or sides of the water container, and do not apply heat directly to the container. Maintain the recommended temperature by adding warm water or removing cool water. The temperature of the water must not be allowed to rise above 112°F (44°C); if it does, serious damage will result. A high-quality thermometer should be used to monitor water temperature. If the body part affected cannot be immersed, hot packs kept within the same temperature range can be applied like compresses; take care, however, not to abrade the skin when applying and removing such packs. An acceptable, but less preferable, alternative to warm water immersion is gradual warming at room temperature.

Two rewarming procedures which should *not* be followed involve the application of snow and ice to the area and the application of excessive heat. The term *excessive heat* refers to temperatures above 120°F (49°C). Radiant heat from hot fires, stoves and vehicle exhaust systems have often been employed by frostbitten victims. So much heat can cause the affected area to burst, splitting the skin and muscle tissue; severe and irreparable damage will result.

As the affected area is rewarmed (properly), the victim will experience pain, the degree of pain varying in proportion to the vitality of the cardiovascular system. Assuming that the victim is in no danger of further exposure to the cold, small quantities of alcohol, sedatives or analgesics may be administered for the often-intolerable pain associated with rewarming.

Once thawed, it is imperative that the affected part be kept clean and dry until medical attention is available.

Three *don'ts* are to be remembered:

1. Don't rub or massage the affected part before, during, or after thawing; this warning applies to the victim as well as the rescuer.

2. Don't allow the victim to risk re-exposure to the cold.

3. Don't allow smoking; smoking causes vasoconstriction which will interfere with the recovery process.

The treatment of fractures and dislocations with frostbite victims is very complicated. Traction, manipulation or tight wrapping of the limbs should be avoided if at all possible. Except in the case of dislocation in mild frostbite cases, it is advisable to leave the injured part alone until medical attention can be obtained.

PREVENTION

While there is no doubt that severe cold and chilling winds are the chief causes of frostbite, many other factors can contribute to it.

Water on the skin or clothing greatly increases the risk of frostbite. Every effort must be made to dry and replace wet clothing in the field, if possible.

Fear, panic, exhaustion and malnutrition can all lead to frostbite in that they encourage inadvisable actions and often reduce the body's resistance to the cold. Frequent rest stops, snacking, light exercise (if needed) and rewarming enroute are strongly recommended. Travel should be with companions and situations avoided which are likely to endanger life. Accidents are one of the leading attendant factors associated with frostbite. The only factor more highly associated with frostbite than accidents is alcoholic intoxication. Alcohol consumption has no place in the severe cold!

The easiest way to prevent frostbite is to dress carefully. Outerwear should be selected which will minimize skin exposure, especially in wet, windy weather. Constricting garments, particularly around the ankles and wrists, should be avoided as they tend to reduce circulation and thus promote cooling. Warm, waterproof gloves, hat, and boots are advisable. Felt liners for boots have become increasingly popular during recent years, but they are not recommended when frostbite is a potential problem. Any moisture reaching the felt, even sweat, is absorbed and the liners will slowly begin to expand. The resulting tightening can inhibit circulation and increase the risk of frostbitten feet.

A comment should also be made in reference to Reynaud's disease and various other diseases which cause impaired circulation in the extremities. These disorders can predispose one to frostbite.

Again, it is recommended that people check each other's faces often when outside in severe cold; early treatment of the symptoms of frostbite can serve to prevent a major problem.

CHAPTER 8

Rewarming, Cardiopulmonary Resuscitation (CPR) and Field Rescue

There is little consensus among physicians and medical researchers regarding the "best" course of treatment for the victim of primary accidental hypothermia. For victims of secondary accidental hypothermia, matters are further complicated by the specific characteristics of the underlying disorder.

For the most part, questions and debates within medical circles hinge on the availability of certain types of equipment, the experience and training of the personnel involved and, ultimately, the professional judgment of the physician in charge. Sophisticated treatment of the hypothermia victim is a relatively recent phenomenon. Although there are many techniques and procedures used for treatment, only a handful of physicians have experience with them; thus there are limited data available for researchers to evaluate. All procedures and techniques about to be discussed have shown reasonable degrees of success under various conditions.

With the exception of the material on rescue and first aid, the medical information presented here is intended for educational purposes only. It is not intended to provide a "do it yourself" guide for treatment of the hypothermia victim.

The reason for this is that even in the best of circumstances a hypothermia victim may have neural, cardiovascular or respiratory complications, and/or blood chemistry disturbances. Given the likelihood of such serious complications, professional medical assistance should be obtained as soon as possible. Once physicians or emergency medical technicians have taken charge of the victim, others should not presume to "second guess" them in their treatment, decisions or recommendations.

While first aid and rescue often fall unavoidably on the shoulders of the medically unsophisticated, clinical treatment of any disorder as serious as hypothermia clearly lies in the realm of the physician. Even victims who may return to a seemingly normal state as a result of first aid in the field should also be seen by medical personnel in order to ascertain that an uncomplicated recovery has indeed taken place.

CARDIOPULMONARY RESUSCITATION

The term cardiopulmonary resuscitation (CPR) is used to describe an emergency lifesaving technique which frequently restores ventilation and heart function in victims of drownings, certain types of cardiac arrests and other accidents or mishaps. Since hypothermia victims often reach a point at which cardiac and breathing functions cease, CPR is considered to be a recommended action when rendering first aid to the victim.

CPR technique involves three basic steps.

1. Checking the respiratory passage for blockage, and extending the neck in preparation for step two.
2. Providing artificial ventilation by "blowing" down the victim's throat; this measure is taken only if spontaneous breathing does *not* occur.
3. Assisting the standstill heart in propelling blood to all parts of the body by externally compressing the chest.

No one is quite certain why external chest compression (ECC) works as it does. It is known that pushing on the chest causes the entire thorax to act as a large pump. Beyond that, the intricacies of ECC are beyond the scope of this book. However, it is important to realize that ECC involves the physical manipulation of the heart (via the thorax) in order to promote the flow of freshly oxygenated blood.

The reason for addressing the question of CPR in a discussion of hypothermia is that the process of delivering external chest compressions to the chest of a hypothermia victim carries with it the possibility of inducing ventricular fibrillation, as explained previously. Recall that every heart has a period of such susceptibility; if a CPR chest compression triggers unanticipated electrical impulses in the unprepared heart, fibrillation can result.

Despite the risk of ventricular fibrillation, there are situations in which CPR might be advisable for a hypothermia victim. Clearly, it is critical for the body to maintain its cardiac functions. Although the cells of the body can exist for a limited time without the heart pumping fresh blood and oxygen to them, this "period of grace" does not extend indefinitely. If the victim is to survive, the heartbeat must be restored.

As seen, the severe hypothermia victim will be in a state of highly depressed metabolism, all organs (including the heart) will be functioning at very low rates, and all organs will be relatively cold physically. Within the cardiovascular system, the heart beat will be slow, blood pressure will be low, and the blood will be highly viscous. The neuroregulatory system will be functioning far below its peak level of efficiency.

Heartbeat may be present at one or two beats *per minute,* or it may have ceased. The hard decisions for the rescuer are whether the victim is in a state of cardiac arrest and, if so, whether to administer CPR. Either way, there are major risks to be considered.

If the victim *is* in a state of cardiac arrest, CPR might revive cardiac and pulmonary functions, thereby increasing the chances for survival.

If the victim is *not* in a state of cardiac arrest and is simply functioning at an abnormally low level, CPR might trigger ventricular fibrillation which, in turn, can cause death.

Yet a third possibility exists: once CPR is started, it must be continued until the victim has recovered or until artificial support can be extended. Because in some field settings help may not arrive for hours, the person (or persons) administering CPR run the risk of exhaustion. In cold weather, the exertion required by sustained delivery of CPR can in itself lead to hypothermia. Determining the right course of action is difficult! Luckily some guidelines exist.

The first step is to ascertain the victim's level of *consciousness*. If there is consciousness, determine whether he or she is breathing easily, or whether there is coughing or other signs of respiratory distress.

Let's assume that the victim is *conscious and not showing any sign of respiratory distress*. Then we ask, is there *shivering*? If so, provide insulation and warmth (with blankets, warm shower or bath, hot tea or hot chocolate) and allow to rest while under constant observation.

If the victim is conscious and breathing easily, but is *not shivering,* simply insulate and cover or place in bed, allowing the body to spontaneously rewarm itself. As before, watch closely for any change in condition.

Now, let's backtrack a bit. Suppose the victim is *conscious,* but *experiencing difficulty in breathing* (coughing, gasping, etc.). He or she may be experiencing a *very rapid heart rate* (tachycardia) or *very rapid breathing* (tachypnoea) and cyanosis. These signs indicate some form of respiratory distress, and ventilation should be assisted and the victim taken to the hospital as soon as possible.

If there is any respiration at all, assume that the heart is working. A person who is breathing, however slow or difficult the effort, is assumed to have a functioning heart. When dealing with hypothermia victims, *a functioning heart is best left alone.*

If the victim is *unconscious,* but breathing, insulate (passive external rewarming) and transport to a hospital as soon as possible. If *unconscious*, but *not breathing*, immediately check for blockage of the respiratory passageway and begin artificial ventilation. While ventilating, check for a pulse in the neck (carotid). If a pulse can be found, continue artificial ventilation and transport to the hospital as soon as possible. If there is no pulse you are faced with another decision. Although there is controversy concerning this "final" stage, the consensus is that if the person is a drowning victim, begin external chest compressions and transport to the hospital. If the person is hypothermic but not a victim of drowning—do not perform external chest compression, but do continue artificial ventilation and transport to the hospital.

Additional factors must be considered before administering CPR. Chief among them are: (1) the probable length of time that will elapse before CPR relief is available; (2) distance and/or time constraints which might delay medical attention; (3) your own health status vis-à-vis the potential for hypothermia affecting you, as the rescuer.

If, in your judgment, CPR relief and medical attention will arrive before you succumb to fatigue or hypothermia, CPR should be initiated.

If assistance is too remote, or if your own health status is deteriorating, CPR should not be started. Under such circumstances, the victim's best odds for survival lie with the cold. His or her metabolic and cardiopulmonary functions may be suppressed to a point from which revival is possible, and you must take that chance rather than risk triggering ventricular fibrillation or complete heart failure (which can be induced by external chest compression) while beyond the reach of medical assistance. To do otherwise could place your own life, as well as that of the victim, in extreme jeopardy.

REWARMING

The term *rewarming* is about as straightforward as one can get. When applied to the hypothermia victim, it refers to the procedures followed in restoring core temperature to 98.6°F (37°C). *Note:* Rewarming procedures assume that the victim has a fully functioning cardiovascular and respiratory system. If there are no signs of a pulse or breathing, the first aid procedures outlined in the above section on CPR should be followed. There is a wide variety of rewarming procedures which have been tried; they range in sophistication from microwave heating to hot tea. Some are more appropriate than others for certain types of victims, some are better understood than others, and some can be undertaken only in well-equipped clinics by specially trained personnel.

The rewarming of the hypothermia victim is *not* normally a quick process. For many victims, returning core temperature to 98.6°F (37°C) is a process which may take three to eight hours, with others requiring up to 24, or even 48, hours. In some cases, rewarming is done rapidly (30 minutes to two hours), but most victims are warmed slowly in order to minimize the risk of additional trauma.

There are three categories of rewarming procedures: passive external, rapid external and active internal.

Passive external rewarming assumes that the body can spontaneously generate sufficient heat to rewarm itself—providing cold stress has been removed. The procedure includes placing the victim on a dry surface which *does not absorb heat*. (Cold ground will drain away more heat than will an air mattress, for example.) Once placed in relatively warm, dry location, the victim is covered with one or more blankets (or a sleeping bag), and a hat or cap is often placed on the head. Ideally, the insulation under the body and the covering over it will retain the heat which the body generates naturally. Shivering is seen as a highly positive sign. However, should shivering cease, make certain that the victim has warmed rather than exhausted himself. If conscious, warm sugary tea or bouillon can be administered slowly. (Don't permit the victim to hold a spoon, cup or bowl; he will be quite clumsy and hot liquid spills can damage highly vulnerable cold skin.)

In clinical settings, researchers have found that even a very cold, unconscious hypothermia victim can generate sufficient heat to raise the core temperature from a few tenths of a degree to one or two degrees Centigrade per hour.

WRAP WARMED CLOTHS AROUND
HEAD, NECK, CHEST, AND GROIN

COVER WITH BLANKETS

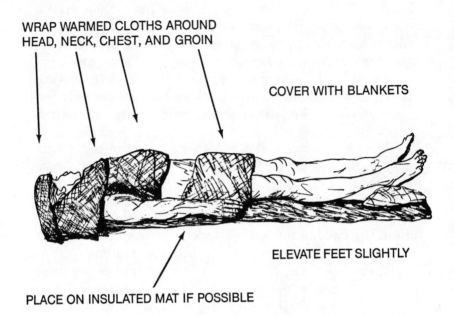

ELEVATE FEET SLIGHTLY

PLACE ON INSULATED MAT IF POSSIBLE

Passive warming includes the use of insultating material under the body, hat or cap, clothing around neck, chest and groin, and one or more blankets.

The critical step is to move the victim to a warm, dry environment shielded from cold stress; once there, the body should be able to recover under its own power.

One of the main physiological advantages of this approach is that it is slow and natural. Remember that the hypothermia victim is often dehydrated, the liver and kidneys not functioning at their normal level, the metabolism severely depressed, the blood not physiologically balanced, and the neuroregulatory systems functioning slowly. When the body is allowed to rewarm slowly, it has the opportunity to coordinate all aspects of recovery so that the "total system" is brought along intact. With the more active approaches, there is always the risk of correcting one subsystem too fast, with the result that certain functions are not synchronized with other, equally critical functions.

Another advantage of the passive approach is that it almost always avoids "rewarming shock," which occurs if the external surface of the extremities warm more rapidly than the core. When this happens, one or more of the following negative effects can result.

1. Rising metabolic rates of cells in the skin and extremities may demand more oxygen and hence more blood than the cold and underactive heart can provide: consequently, those tissues will experience oxygen shortages and acidiosis, an acidic condition of the blood. *Normally,* this condition is neutralized by the blood itself.

2. Heart rate may be more stimulated by the autonomic nervous system than the heart tissue can handle, inducing cardiac arrhythmias.

3. Vasodilatation of the peripheral blood vessels may cause a sudden drop in blood pressure, which would temporarily cause less blood to go to the brain and other vital organs and thus compromise their functions. For this reason it is always wise to warm the victim while in a horizontal position.

Rapid external rewarming, as a category of procedures, includes those techniques which aggressively direct heat to the hypothermia victim's external body surfaces. The term *rapid* is somewhat misleading since some of these techniques may be extended for periods as long as 12–18 hours. *The critical factor is that heat generating sources other than the victim's own are brought into play.*

The most common procedure involves a bathtub, hot tub or whirlpool bath with warm water. This technique may involve immersion of the trunk and limbs, or just the trunk of the body.

Heat cradles are used in some hospitals. These shell-like devices are placed over the victim's trunk and radiant heat is directed toward the cold body. Diathermy and microwave warming techniques employ high-frequency energy waves directed at the body to generate heat in the victim's trunk. Neck coils are specially adapted heating pads intended to warm the neck and, more important, the central areas of the brain stem (including the hypothalamus). Liquid-heated suits through which warm liquid is circulated, like those used more and more by deep-sea divers, have been experimented with in rewarming hypothermia victims. Somewhat similar in approach is the water bed which, when filled with warm water, has been useful in warming some victims.

Many of these techniques are obviously best administered by well-equipped medical facilities. One other technique exists, however, which is useful in the field and which has a long, proven record of success is simple body-to-body contact. Such warming is technically a rapid external approach. While one person can extend some body heat to the hypothermia victim, body-to-body rewarming works best if two or more people are in a sleeping bag or wrapped in blankets with the hypothermia victim. When several "warmers" are used, there is a reduced risk of significant heat loss to the cold body of the victim; all warmers should periodically exercise to warm their own bodies.

Among physicians who recommend the more rapid external approaches, the rationale usually is that in certain circumstances, rapid rewarming reduces the risks of cardiovascular problems, particularly for the very cold [less than 86°F (30°C)] hypothermia victim. While many successful recoveries have been attributed to rapid external rewarming techniques, the evidence that the procedures significantly reduce cardiovascular risks is not decisive; nonetheless, when employed properly, they certainly have their place in the treatment of the hypothermia victim.

The third category of techniques is called active internal rewarming. These techniques are used in highly critical situations, most commonly those in which the victim is *known* to be in a state of cardiovascular collapse. Since death rapidly follows cessation of cardiovascular and cerebral activity, it is imperative that cardiac functions be restored as quickly as possible. Drugs and electroshock are the only available techniques for reactivating the silenced heart, but unfortunately, neither drugs nor electrical stimulation will restore cardiac function unless the heart tissue is above

86°F (30°C). In such circumstances, physicians will often resort to what appear at first glance to be rather drastic measures.

Extracorporeal cardiopulmonary bypass is a technique which involves "tapping" into the vein which runs from the lungs to the heart. There chilled blood is diverted into a machine which contributes a small increment of heat and returns it to the heart for distribution to other parts of the body. As the total blood volume begins to warm, the temperature is gradually raised to 98.6°F (37°C).

On some occasions, warm blood plasma solutions are fed intravenously into the victim. The procedure warms in a manner similar to that of the cardiopulmonary bypass method.

Peritoneal dialysis involves surgically opening the abdominal cavity and placing warm physiologic solutions into it. The procedure serves to warm certain critical organs as well as the blood (which is passing through the arteries and veins in the abdominal cavity). A similar procedure is called *mediastinal lavage*. In this case, warm fluids are circulated through the cavity which cradles the heart.

Intragastric lavage is accomplished by circulating warm fluids through the stomach. At times this involves a direct flushing of the stomach, and at others a balloon is inserted into the stomach and the fluid is circulated through this internalized "hot water bottle."

One of the newest internal rewarming procedures is called *inhalation rewarming*. Warm humidified air (sometimes with a higher than normal concentration of oxygen) is placed into the victim's thorax via the respiratory structures (bronchial tubes, lungs, etc.). This technique is quite promising since it does not require surgery and thus reduces the risk to the victim. Also, the equipment needed is portable, inexpensive and easy to use. For these reasons, the technique may soon become the standard technique for qualified field rescue teams.

As has been mentioned, all of the above techniques have been used successfully, just as all have had their share of failures. It would appear, with the exception of those instances in which there is clearcut evidence indicating cardiovascular collapse, that any one of these techniques stands an equal chance of success. *Passive external rewarming is undoubtedly the safest approach for the medically inexperienced person who must undertake rewarming of a victim.*

A topic that deserves to be discussed in reference to rewarming is *afterdrop*. This is a phenomenon often recorded in clinical settings, but because it involves monitoring core temperature via the rectum, it is seldom observed in the field by nonmedical personnel.

Afterdrop refers to the fact that once rewarming has been initiated and core temperature has started to rise, a sudden drop in core temperature will often occur. After this short drop, the temperature will then resume its climb. For many years, it was thought that this was a phenomenon peculiar to hypothermic humans and that it was what triggered ventricular fibrillation. *It has subsequently been determined that it is simply a function of the body's normal response to rewarming.* In warming hypothermia victims, more attention should be paid to cardiovascular and respiratory integrity and less to afterdrop.

Such complications and deaths as do occur during rewarming are usually due to some underlying disease condition. Such disorders cannot, in most cases, be anticipated or treated by the layman, and the *passive external approach allows the body its best chance at physiological self-regulation and self-preservation.* In many, if not most rescue situations, competent medical assistance will become available before passive rewarming has run its full course. When it arrives, such medical intervention as may be needed can be provided without undue risk to the victim.

A WORD ABOUT ALCOHOL

Alcohol has been used in efforts to rewarm cold people for thousands of years. The use of St. Bernard Dogs for locating and rescuing lost travelers in the Swiss Alps is a classical example of this approach. What most people don't know is that the little kegs carried by the dogs contained a sugar solution which was lightly laced with brandy. Straight brandy, or any other alcoholic beverage, causes only superficial warming. The blood vessels near the skin vasodilate, thus creating the sensation of heat. Such vaso-dilation requires increased blood flow to the skin and the heart must work harder by increasing its rate to provide that extra flow. Initially, if the heart can't meet the new demand, unconsciousness is a likely result, but more serious car-diovascular complications are possible.

A second danger from alcohol stems from the fact that the vasodilation process signals to the thermal receptors that the skin is warming. The receptors, in turn, lower the urgency of the alert they are sending to the thermoregula-tory center. Shivering is thereby suppressed and a powerful mechanism for heat production is lost.

Alcohol is *not* recommended as a part of the rewarming process, then, since it may mask the symptoms of hypother-mia and interfere with the body's normal recuperative func-tions. The victim might look and feel warm, but inside the cold core will remain untouched by life-giving warmth and, in fact, may continue to lose what little heat remains.

RESCUE

Because of the many different situations in which one is liable to encounter hypothermia, this brief section is de-signed to offer only general guidelines for the very first steps to be taken upon discovering a hypothermia victim. (Note, however, that rescuers of water-related accident victims should be familiar with the material contained in Chapter 6.) The assumption is made here that the rescuer is medi-cally untrained and has no special rescue or physiological monitoring equipment available, including a thermometer. For those who have special medical or first aid training as well as access to field monitoring equipment, treatment procedures above and beyond those discussed here may be appropriate. Several references listed at the end of the book are suggested for further reading.

A major recommendation is to be alert constantly for

hypothermia's warning signs in yourself and in those with you. Rescue should *start* the minute hypothermia warning signs appear. Waiting only increases the problems to be faced and decreases the victim's chances of survival.

Keep your eyes open for the following symptoms:

Excellent.

1. Continual shivering.
2. Poor coordination.
3. Slowing of pace; hanging back.
4. Increasingly numb hands and feet. This leads to stumbling, clumsiness and loss of dexterity.
5. Dazed confused behavior; victim may be careless and forgetful.
6. Speech slurred and slow; slow to respond to questions.
7. Hallucinations.
8. Pupils dilated.
9. Decreased attention span.

If any of these signs appear, it's time to begin rewarming procedures. To wait even 15–20 minutes may be too long. If you respond to the early symptoms in time, your chances of beating hypothermia are quite good. The longer you delay, the poorer your chances become.

Every hypothermia victim is a candidate for passive external rewarming. This statement holds true for the elderly in a cold home or apartment, the deep-sea diver who has been submerged too long, the backpacker caught in a chilling storm, or the mountain climber trapped by a blizzard. Whether the victim is superficially or severely affected, the following objectives are recommended as first aid. (When drowning or near-drowning is involved, drowning aspects must be addressed before those associated with hypothermia.)

1. *Prevent further heat loss.*

a. Remove wet or cold clothing and dry the victim. If necessary, cut clothing off of the victim in order to reduce physical abuse in the effort to remove garments. If only passive external rewarming is to be employed (see below), reclothe the victim in warm, dry clothing. Use several layers if possible; use a hat or cap for the head and a scarf around the neck.

b. Move the victim into some sort of warmer, protective shelter. It is very important to *insulate the victim* from the weather, including rain, snow, wind and other drafts, and from the earth.

2. *Avoid manhandling the victim.* Jostling or rolling the victim around may produce undesirable physical shocks to the internal organs. Be as gentle as possible.

3. *Seek medical assistance* if it is possible to do so without endangering the life of anyone in the party, including the victim. Be especially aware of additional hypothermia cases. If one member of a group has fallen prey to hypothermia, others may soon follow. Rewarm everyone before sending for help.

4. *Rewarm the victim.* If the victim is conscious:

a. Encourage movement (if shivering is not yet pronounced) *unless* the size of the available shelter prevents it; *shelter is more important than movement at this point.*

b. Slowly feed the victim hot, sugary tea, hot chocolate or bouillon. [About 110°F (42°C) is right—just slightly warm to the touch.]

c. Wrap the victim in a sleeping bag or several blankets.

d. Try to keep the victim awake and talking.

e. Keep the victim's head at least level with the body; some slight elevation of the legs and feet is desirable.

f. Wrap a scarf over the victim's mouth. This will help retain body heat while it also warms incoming air.

g. In an open situation move as many people as possible into the shelter so that their body heat can warm the victim's immediate environment. Warm rocks or a fire (at a distance) will also help raise "local" temperature.

If the victim is unconscious, no effort should be made to force warm liquids into the throat. [Cardiopulmonary resuscitation (CPR) *may* be indicated; refer to the section on CPR for guidelines.]

If the victim is semiconscious or unconscious, nothing more active than the above procedures is recommended. If the victim is still able to shiver [core temperature is above 89.6°F (32°C)], then more active rewarming procedures may be employed. A cautionary note is in order: *Do not proceed with active rewarming techniques unless you have good reason to believe that the signs and symptoms observed in the victim are due to hypothermia and not to some underlying disorder.*

Here are several active external rewarming techniques which can be easily employed in field rescue situations if you are confident more aggressive procedures are needed.

1. Body-to-body contact. The victim and one or preferably two "warmers" should be nude rather than clothed or wearing only undergarments. Whenever possible, at least one, but preferably two or more sleeping bags should be used. The more that can be done to conserve body heat, the better. A hat on the head and a scarf around the victim's neck are highly desirable. The victim should lie between the two warmers arranged to provide maximum skin-to-skin contact. If enough people are available, the warmers should be relieved after approximately 30 minutes. All warmers should exercise vigorously before starting their rewarming attempt and afterward to maintain their own temperatures.

2. Warm bath or hot tub (showers are much less desirable). This approach *must* be used *only* with a conscious victim. Water should be approximately 70°F (20°C) when starting out; after 10–20 minutes, it may be raised gradually to 110°F (42°C).

3. Warm compresses. Hot water bottles [up to 110°F (42°C)], warm rocks wrapped in towels or blankets, heated towels, warm water-filled canteens, etc. can be used in this approach. The heated compresses or containers are wrapped around or are placed next to the trunk of the victim.

One active *internal* rewarming procedure which can be successfully employed in the field is mouth-to-mouth respiration. Breathing into the respiratory passages of the victim forces warm air into the chest cavity; both the warmth and the oxygen supplied are helpful to the victim. This technique is a modification of the inhalation rewarming method discussed earlier. Mouth-to-mouth respiration should not be employed if it causes panic on the part of the victim or if it interferes with the respiratory processes.

Several other points must be mentioned in reference to rescue procedures.

1. Never leave the conscious victim alone if avoidable.

2. Don't transport the victim if it seems likely that medical assistance can be brought to the victim. Transportation increases the likelihood of physical stress and shock.

3. Never administer alcohol to a hypothermia victim.

4. Encourage the conscious victim to consume as much *warm* liquid as possible; include sugar or honey if possible.

5. Do not give the victim any sedatives, tranquilizers, pain killers, aspirin, or other medications.

6. Do not massage, rub or jostle the victim.

7. Do not permit smoking. Smoking causes vasoconstriction which retards blood flow to the hands and feet as well as to the skin.

8. During rescue efforts, shield the victim from windchills caused by boat, truck, snowmobile or other modes of transportation, and from helicopter blades.

CHAPTER 9

Preventing Hypothermia

Hypothermia is one of the most insidious dangers to strike the unsuspecting and the unprepared. Water at a temperature below 98.6°F (37°C) will take away body heat at a rate 25 times faster than air will, and that doesn't take into account the temperature difference between the body and the water. Cold wet clothing literally refrigerates the body, and people have been known to suffer hypothermia at temperatures well above freezing. Men and women have been known to survive for a month or more without food, and for at least a week without water, but placed in a situation where heat loss is continual, a person may succumb within hours.

With the possible exception of accidental injuries, there is seldom any excuse for a person to become hypothermic. We must understand our bodies and any limitations imposed by personal health. We must also understand the environment and its vagaries. Having that knowledge gives one an almost intuitive awareness of defensive capabilities in the face of circumstances which might upset thermal balance. Add to that the body's sophisticated thermal detection and warning system, and we are in good shape . . . if we are wise enough to listen to the danger signals.

142

PREVENTION ON THE LAND

Even though the literature of exploration and adventure is filled with accounts of people freezing to death, most such tragic occurrences could have been avoided. People have been known to survive airplane crashes in the Arctic for as many as sixty days because they kept their wits about them and were aware of the rules for wilderness survival.

The following recommendations apply to anyone going beyond the *immediate* reach of civilization, and while they are somewhat oriented toward persons who are traveling, or who are engaging in recreational sports, they apply equally well to those working in severe weather, frequently in isolated locations.

Always File a Complete Travel Plan

An essential rule for all travelers is to keep friends or relatives advised of travel plans. Leave a written record of expected route, destination and arrival time. Include the names, ages and addresses of all members of the party. Specify any known health problems and medication requirements. A list of supplies and survival equipment should be attached to the travel plan. If the trip includes check points from which updated information, changes and progress reports can be filed, do it.

Be Aware of Weather Forecasts

Reference to *snow* in a National Weather Service forecast, without a qualification such as *occasional* or *intermittent,* means that anticipated fall is of a steady nature and will probably continue for several hours without letup.

Snow flurries are defined as snow falling for short durations at intermittent periods; flurries may reduce visibilities to an eighth of a mile or less. Accumulations from snow flurries are generally small.

Snow squalls are brief, intense falls of snow and are comparable to summer rain showers. They are accompanied by gusty surface winds.

Blowing and drifting snow generally occur together and are a result of strong winds and falling snow or loose snow on the gound. *Blowing snow* is defined as snow lifted from the surface by the wind and blown about to a degree that horizontal visibility is greatly restricted. *Drifting snow* is used in forecasts to indicate that strong winds will blow falling snow or loose snow on the ground into significant drifts. In the northern plains, the combination of blowing and drifting snow, *after* a substantial snowfall has ended, is often referred to as a *ground blizzard.*

Blizzards are the most dramatic and perilous of all winter storms, characterized by strong winds bearing large amounts of snow. Most of the snow accompanying a blizzard is in the form of fine, powdery particles whipped in such great quantities that at times visibility is only a few yards.

The National Weather Service issues the following watches and warnings for *hazardous* winter weather events.

Winter Storm Watch
Severe winter weather conditions may affect your area.

Winter Storm Warning
Severe winter weather conditions are *imminent.*

Ice Storm Warning
Significant, possibly damaging, ice accumulation is expected. Freezing rain (or drizzle) means precipitation is expected to freeze when it hits exposed surfaces.

Heavy Snow Warning
A snowfall of at least 4 inches in 12 hours or 6 inches in 24 hours is expected. (Heavy snow can mean lesser amounts where winter storms are infrequent.)

Blizzard Warning
Considerable falling and/or blowing snow and winds of at least 35 miles per hour, and temperatures of 20°F or lower are expected for several hours.

Severe Blizzard Warning

Considerable falling and/or blowing snow, winds of at least 45 miles per hour, and temperatures of 10°F or lower are expected for several hours.

High Wind Warning

Winds of at least 40 miles per hour are expected to last for at least 1 hour. (In some areas, this means strong gusty winds occurring in shorter time periods.)

Always Carry a Survival Kit

Survival kits are *emergency* supplies which should be carried in addition to other supplies. They should be used only in an emergency. Commercial kits varying in complexity and usefulness are available from outdoor equipment suppliers, sporting goods dealers and some mail order companies. Many survival handbooks listed in the Selected Reading section at the end of this book contain recommendations for assembling the type of kit needed for various situations. Evaluate your needs and develop a kit that will help *you* save *your life.*

A minimum, short-term survival kit (such as one carried in an automobile) might include:

Boy Scout or Swiss Army style knife
9 × 12 ft plastic tarp with grommets
50 ft of nylon rope
3-gal can (for cooking, melting snow)
tea bags
boullion cubes
chocolate
honey or sugar cubes
candles
adhesive tape
flashlight
stiff wire (for use as a bucket bail, etc.)
large trash bags (quick waterproof shelter)
waterproof matches
signal flare and signal flag

small change for pay phone
first aid kit
whistle
a good survival handbook

More extensive kits include larger quantities of the above items as well as the following items.

water purification tablets
toilet paper
sanitary napkins
sunglasses with case
sun protection lotion
smoke signals
large machete or hand axe
camp stove with fuel
3–5 days of trail rations
maps and compass
fishing gear, snares, etc.
mirror for signaling
shovel
sack of sand
booster cables
tow chains
catalytic heater
fire extinguisher
paper towels

Remember: survival kits are useful only if they are handy (and complete) when you need them.

Never Travel Alone Unless it is Absolutely Necessary

Ask yourself if it *is* absolutely necessary.

Wear, or at Least Carry, Clothing Suitable for the Worst Weather You Could Expect

Survival texts recommend that you layer clothing so

that garments can be added or removed quickly and easily, according to the demands of the weather and your level of exertion. Wool is strongly recommended because it is able to retain some heat even when wet and it dries quickly. Cotton is a very poor insulating fabric when wet and it dries slowly.

Always carry a *spare* woolen watch cap, high-quality gloves, a windbreaker and a scarf or breathing mask. The importance of good waterproof boots cannot be overstated. If your clothing gets wet, stop and dry it *immediately!* Use a fire, slap wet clothes against a tree, do whatever is necessary to dry your garments.

Make Camp Early

Even if you are carrying your own tent for shelter, setting up a weather-secure camp takes time and energy. If the weather is severe, even more time and energy will be required. Stopping early ensures that you won't be rushed by nightfall and you'll be less likely to make mistakes or overlook important safety points. You'll be fresh enough to think clearly.

Hypothermia sneaks up on its victims: a fatigued camper trying to set up camp may fail to rig the tent properly, which leads to water in the tent, which leads to wet clothing and sleeping bags, which leads to . . .

Allow time and the energy to do things right.

Know How to Construct an Emergency Shelter

A good survival handbook will show how to build a lean-to or snow shelter. It will also illustrate ways to take advantage of "natural shelter," such as fallen trees. Memorize those techniques! Even a "quickie" shelter can take hours to construct if you are cold and wet. Consider the use of tube tents, plastic tarps, plastic leaf bags and other items that can be used for emergency shelter with a minimum amount of exertion.

Don't Fight Storms

The only animal known to wander around in severe storms is man; not even polar bears pit themselves against the fury of the elements unnecessarily. Very few scheduled "appointments" are worth risking hypothermia. Better to spend a few hours, or days, holed up safely than to endanger your life trying to keep a schedule.

If you sense a storm coming up:

1. get into your storm gear before you get wet; and
2. make and take shelter immediately.

In wind, rain, and cold, hypothermia can be fatal before morning. All you have to do is give it a chance to get started. Protect yourself and ride out bad weather.

The National Oceanic and Atmospheric Administration (NOAA) advises all persons to prepare for winter storms with the following steps.

1. *Keep ahead of winter storms* by listening to the latest weather warnings and bulletins on radio and television.

2. *Check battery-powered equipment* before a storm arrives. A portable radio or television set may be your only contact with the world outside. Also check emergency cooking facilities and flashlights.

3. *Check your supply of heating fuel.* Fuel carriers may not be able to move if a winter storm buries an area in snow.

4. *Check your food* and stock an extra supply. Supplies should include food that requires no cooking or refrigeration in the event of power failure.

5. *Prevent fire hazards* due to overheated coal or oil burning stoves, fireplaces, heaters, or furnaces. Be sure to provide a constant replacement of oxygen depleted by a heat source.

6. *Stay indoors during storms* and cold snaps unless in peak physical condition. If you must go out, avoid overexertion.

7. *Don't kill yourself shoveling snow.* It is extremely hard work for anyone in less than prime physical condition,

and can bring on a heart attack, a major cause of death during and after winter storms.

8. *Rural residents.* Make necessary trips for supplies before a storm develops or not at all: arrange for emergency heat supply in case of power failure: be sure camp stoves and lanterns are fueled.

9. *Dress to fit the season.* If you spend much time outdoors, wear loose fitting, lightweight, warm clothing in several layers that can be removed to prevent perspiring and subsequent chill. Outer garments should be tightly woven, water repellent, and hooded. The hood should protect much of the face and cover the mouth to ensure warm breathing and protect the lungs from the extremely cold air. Remember that entrapped, insulating air, warmed by body heat, is the best protection against cold. Layers of relatively light protective clothing are more effective and efficient than a single layer of thick clothing. Mittens, snug at the wrist, are better protection than fingered gloves.

10. *An automobile can be your best friend—or worst enemy—during winter storms,* depending on your preparations. Have your car winterized before the storm season begins. Everything on the following checklist should be taken care of *before* winter storms strike your area.

   ignition system
   battery
   lights
   tire tread
   cooling system
   fuel system
   lubrication
   heater
   brakes adjusted
   wiper blades
   defroster
   snow tires installed
   chains
   antifreeze
   exhaust system tight
   winter grade oil

Keep water out of the fuel system by maintaining a *full* tank, and by occasionally adding "dry gas."

11. *Be prepared for the worst.* Carry a winter storm car kit, especially if cross-country travel is anticipated or if you live in the northern states.

12. *Winter travel by automobile is serious business.* Take your travel seriously.

If the storm exceeds or even tests your limitations, seek available refuge immediately.

Plan your travel and select primary and alternate routes.

Check latest weather information on your radio.

Try not to travel alone; two or three persons are preferable.

Travel in convoy with another vehicle if possible.

Always fill the fuel tank before entering open country, even for a short distance.

Drive carefully, defensively.

Avoid the Use of Alcohol

Alcohol accelerates heat loss, desensitizes the body's thermal detection system and fouls your self-protection mechanisms. It can also lead to unwise and even foolish survival behavior.

Avoid Smoking

Tobacco causes vasoconstriction, which reduces blood flow to the skin, hands and feet. There is a resultant stress on the heart and an increased risk of frostbite.

Conserve and Replenish Energy

Think before you act. Don't perform unnecessary tasks. Be certain rations include both short- and long-term energy resources. Take frequent breaks for sugary tea and rest. Don't underestimate the need for *warm* liquids while in the cold; dehydration can be a real problem. Don't push or over exert yourself. "Fatigue is hypothermia's stepping stone."

Avoid Working Up a Sweat and Stay Dry

Work and travel slowly. Sweating leads to evaporation and evaporation is one of the fastest ways of cooling the human body.

Beware of Wind Chill and Frostbite

Keep aware of early warning signs of frostbite and hypothermia—constantly. Check yourself and the other members of your party for them frequently.

Stay Together

Never allow members of your party to become separated along the trail. There is greater safety in numbers, even when the only enemy is the weather.

Keep in Contact with Others ·

If you are working outside in severe weather, have a pre-set schedule for checking in with other workers, headquarters or someone else

If you are working in an isolated situation, take the precautions you would take if you were camping alone. Don't take chances or think you are exempt from danger just because you're "on the job."

Build a Fire

It may be necessary for warmth and for signaling. Don't build a fire under a tree where a pile of melted snow may suddenly drench it. Don't waste time trying to get a fire started until you have a shelter set up. In severe weather, shelter is more crucial than a fire.

Use Isometric Exercises to Keep Muscles Flexible and to Generate Body Heat

Avoid active exercises that "pump" air through your clothes.

PREVENTION ON THE WATER

Boating and aircraft accidents often leave people afloat, exposed to both wind and water. Unlike their counterparts on land, persons afloat often have little in the way of natural resources to help them. Review those recommendations for prevention of hypothermia on land—many of the same principles apply on the water as well. For example, always file a travel plan, avoid traveling alone, avoid alcohol and smoking, etc.

Have Life Jackets Available

If life jackets are not worn aboard at all times, keep them stowed in a handy location known to all passengers. Flotation jackets are preferable to life vests. Good jackets which cover the waist and groin may double survival time in the water because of their insulating characteristics.

Beware of the Wind

On the open sea, the wind can be as chilling as the water. Even on sunny days, it can easily rob the body of warmth. Boaters, like other outdoors people, are advised to wear layered clothing which they can adjust according to environmental conditions. Wool shirts and sweaters are highly recommended. Good-quality windbreakers, preferably with drawstring hoods and waistbands are a must on board. Wool watch caps cannot be beat for heat retention.

Keep Storm Gear Handy

Make certain all passengers know where this equipment is stowed; put it on *before* you get wet. Treat sea spray and waves with the respect you give to a chilling rain—all promote heat loss.

Carry a Survival Kit

Always carry a survival kit adequate for the number of people on board. All passengers should know where it is stowed. Even small fishing craft should carry some sort of survival equipment. In addition, *make certain at least two people on board are able to operate the vessel.*

The following recommendations pertain to those who find themselves *in* the water.

Be Aware of Warm Water as Well as Cold

Any water that is below skin temperature will drain heat, and hypothermia is known even in tropical waters. Many are soon chilled by 75°F (24°C) water.

Don't Panic If You Suddenly Find Yourself Immersed

Frantic movement, including senseless swimming, does nothing except waste energy.

Stay with Your Vessel

Stay with it, that is unless it is burning or sinking. Most capsized boats will remain afloat, and some will ride high enough out of the water to allow a fairly dry retreat.

Keep Your Shoes On

Shoes will conserve valuable heat, and you will need them when you reach land or are rescued. The only exception to this rule is if you are trying to swim without some sort of flotation device, in which case, they will become a weight liability and should be removed.

Shark Bags Can Help Prevent Hypothermia

Johnson Bag Shark Protectors resemble floating trash bags with a cork life ring at the mouth, and offer some protection against sharks. By staying inside you can reduce exposure to the more turbulent water on the outside.

Stay Clothed

If possible, work your hands up into the sleeves of your jacket; keep your face away from the wind and waves; use your hat and hood; take advantage of every drawstring available. The more you can do to shield your body from the cold water, the better your chances for survival.

Try to Keep Your Party Together

In the water, huddle together in a circle; doing so will help morale and will conserve energy and body warmth.

Take Your Survival Kit with You

Oddly, many people abandon ship and leave their survival equipment behind. If the kit isn't stowed with the life raft, make certain it goes overboard with you. It helps if the kit floats.

Life Raft Procedures

If you are in a life raft, rig a shield against the wind, and dry your clothes immediately if possible. If you have been in the water and manage to get into a raft or to the shore, eat some rations. You will need glucose and other energy resources to rewarm your body. Huddling in the raft will also help.

CHAPTER 10

Hypothermia As A Friend

Up to this point in our examination of hypothermia, the cold has generally been cast in the role of villain. Subnormal body temperatures aren't always threatening, however, and in fact, there are any number of ways in which hypothermia serves useful purposes.

The use of cold as an aid in the treatment of high fevers and various other maladies has a long and often picturesque history. One such application stems from the Crusades when, in the year 1192, Richard the Lion-Hearted and the Sultan Saladin were engaged in fierce combat. Both men, and their armies, were ruthless, but as often happens, they also had great respect for each other. When Saladin heard that Richard was ill with a very high fever, the Turkish warrior sent an emmissary bearing fresh pears and peaches, as well as several tubs of snow. Saladin's personal physician accompanied the gifts and once in Richard's camp, he personally supervised packing the English king in the snow, thereby cooling his body until the fever had subsided.

In a similar manner, the ancient Chinese physician Ch-Hua t'o frequently used icy water from a garden trough to treat patients afflicted with high fevers. The Egyptians, too, are known to have used cold to assist in the curing of diseases at least as early as 2,500 B.C.

In more modern times, Dr. William Wright instituted a treatment center in Liverpool, England between 1776 and 1797, in which he employed cold water baths. James Currie, a Scottish physician, used cold to lower body temperatures in the treatment of disease in 1792, and Baron Dominique Jean Larrey, Napoleon's physician, had the damaged arms and legs of wounded soldiers packed in snow prior to amputation as the best anesthetic available. Throughout the late 1800s, cold was used for a variety of medical purposes, but relatively little systematic data were collected, and there was no rigorous evaluation of the practices then in vogue. In general, the medical community's reception of the cold as a part of the treatment regimen was, if you'll pardon the expression, lukewarm.

In the late 1930s, hypothermia was first used in treating cancer and neuropsychiatric patients. Those early clinical reports on the effects of cold on the body prompted several Nazi physicians to "experiment" on eight inmates of the concentration camps at Dachau. Experiment is a term too kind for their efforts, since the inmates were simply exterminated by prolonged exposure to 39.2°F (4°C) water. However, for the first time, systematic data were collected.

Starting in the 1940s and continuing to the present, the cold has gained widespread acceptance as an important clinical tool in the practice of medicine. *Cold body temperatures in and of themselves do not "cure" diseases or increase healing, but they do reduce certain stresses on the body and they slow down the overall metabolic processes.* Often these changes enable various medications and techniques to work more efficiently and allow the body to devote more of its resources to "self-healing" and less to its normal maintenance functions.

One of the chief benefits to be had from the cold has been its role in the preservation of blood for blood banks. Fresh blood can be stored in a usable form for only 21 days, but as cold-technology was developed for freezing and thawing supplies, blood shelf-life was extended almost indefinitely. Previously, literally thousands of pints of blood were wasted each year as a result of spoilage; now, even the most exotic of blood types can be stored for ready access.

A vast amount of open-heart and other cardiovascular surgery is performed using hypothermia as an essential tool in the process. In such surgery, the blood is circulated through a heart–lung bypass machine which supplies adequate oxygen levels. It also cools the blood, thus inducing and maintaining a core temperature at subnormal level. This procedure is much faster than whole-body cooling and is so efficient that a core temperature of 59°F (15°C) can be attained in 30–45 minutes. Because the cold so drastically reduces the oxygen requirements of the brain and the cardiovascular system, a surgeon can enter the heart, correct any one of a number of problems and then repair the incisions. This use of hypothermia also increases blood viscosity, which allows surgery on organs with high blood flow.

The body's reduced oxygen requirements also make hypothermia an important aid in treating certain lung problems, neurologic disorders, severe kidney failure, heat stroke and fever, in organ transplant surgery, and in treating certain types of tumors.

In recent years, the evolution of microsurgery has also utilized hypothermia. This is a highly sophisticated area of medicine in which the instruments used are very small and delicate. Using this "ultra-fine" equipment, a surgeon, working with powerful magnifying lenses, is able to repair tiny blood vessels, nerves and other minute tissues, and to reattach fingers, hands, feet and even arms severed from the body.

In reattaching appendages of the body it has been found that packing the severed part in ice and cooling the traumatized portion of the body itself reduces the extent of permanent damage and vastly increases the likelihood of success. The story is told of a small boy from South Dakota who had heard about microsurgery on television only a few days before his father had a hand cut off in an accident. The boy reportedly insisted that his father's hand be packed in ice and taken along to the hospital, where microsurgery was performed. The father eventually was able to regain full function of his hand and returned to his profession—an eye doctor.

Within the fields of agriculture, biology and zoology, many research and development efforts are in progress for extending the use of freezing artificial insemination and for preserving various animal life forms. Commercial laboratories are being operated in many states for the purpose of storing human and other types of animal sperm cells, particularly those of beef cattle. In the case of cattle, frozen semen has been thawed and used successfully after being stored for several years. Freezing of beef embryos is not as easily managed, although short-term survival is typically accomplished in about 25% of those frozen. Scientists are confident that the technology for long-term storage of sperm, ova and embryos will become available within the next decade, and they are storing the germ cells of any endangered species at $-384°F$ $(-231.1°C)$ in the expectation that techniques for successful thawing will be developed in the near future. It is hoped new populations of these endangered species can be promoted in this manner.

When such attempts are made to preserve life, the tissue is first bathed in special cryogenic solutions because all cells contain water, as well as other fluids, and freezing them causes the formation of ice crystals. These crystals ordinarily would rupture the cell membranes, thus causing permanent damage, but cryogenic solutions draw out some of the cell's water, help protect the cell membranes, and provide a fairly stable environment for the cell. The cooling process typically involves lowering the temperature at a rate of $1.8°F$ $(1°C)$ per minute until the desired storage temperature is reached.

Sea urchins and fertilized rat, mouse and rabbit embryos have been frozen and have been revived to their normal state. There is a report of a British scientist who froze and revived a golden hamster. Thus far, however, no other multicellular organism has been successfully frozen, thawed and fully revitalized. While there has been only nominal success in the freezing and revival of complex organisms, many look to the day when cold-induced "suspended anima-tion" will be used to "hold" terminally ill patients until some future age when a cure for their disease is developed.

Meanwhile, there is a worldwide Cryonics Society which stores "dead" patients in "solid state hypothermia," although many members of the society have had their bodies frozen at death, most scientists are quite skeptical about the odds for successful revival. On the other hand, promoters of cryogenics argue that even a slim chance at post-death revi-val offers better odds than embalming and burial. They believe that future technology will be equal to the challeng-ing tasks of revival and return to life. They acknowledge that the "frozen dead" cannot be revived with present methods, but believe that there is always hope.

Such visions as these do offer hope, however, one may judge their prospects for fulfillment. Hypothermia can be a friend, and an agent in healing; for most of us, most of the time, however, cold is but another of nature's elements, a force with which we must contend in daily life. Still, it is hoped that the information contained in this book will help in coping more effectively with cold.

Keep warm!

Appendix

Emergency Treatment of Hypothermia

G. Patrick Lilja, M.D.

Director of Trauma and Emergency Medicine
North Memorial Medical Center
Minneapolis, Minnesota

Must suspect hypothermia to diagnose. Remember—in severe hypothermia patient may appear dead.

I. Diagnose Degree of Hypothermia
   A. Mild: 97°F–95°F (35°C–34°C)
   B. Moderate: 94°F–86°F (34°C–30°C)
   C. Severe: less than 86°F (30°C)

II. Hospital Management—depends on degree of hypothermia present. Must have "low reading" *rectal* thermometer.
   A. Mild
      1. Externally warm the patient, using either warm blankets, heat lamp or warm fluids.

163

2. Check for frostbite.
3. Check for a predisposing factor (underlying pathology).
B. Moderate and severe
   1. Assure adequate airway; if unconscious gently intubate.
   2. If there is no pulse, begin cardiopulmonary resuscitation. Start intravenous infusion with Ringers lactate prewarmed to 107°F (42°C).
   3. Draw appropriate blood samples; for example, check for glucose, blood urea nitrogen toxicology, blood gases, complete blood counts, electrolytes (usually sodium, potassium chloride, and carbon dioxide).
   4. Start central venous pressure line and monitor central venous pressure closely. Maintain adequate fluid volume as patient warms—*this is a must.*
   5. Start on humidified, heated oxygen 102°F–112°F (40°C–44°C).
   6. Catheterize the patient, using a Foley catheter.
   7. Begin rewarming procedure (basic principles to remember):
      a. Watch fluid status as patient warms, including frequent central venous pressure and blood pressure checks. Give fluid to maintain adequate circulation.
      b. Correct blood gases for temperature; some acidosis is desirable.
      c. Do not use antibiotics.
      d. Do not treat hyperglycemia while rewarming unless so severe that patient is hyperosmolar.
      e. If patient is in cardiac arrest continue cardiopulmonary resuscitation until warm.
   8. Definitive treatment (rewarming) for moderate and severe hypothermia
      a. If core temperature is 93°F–86°F (34°C–30°C) use:

1. Heated, humidified oxygen through face mask if available.
2. Radiant heat—using heat lamps such as those from a nursery for newborns.
3. Warm tub *with caution* (it is difficult to monitor—if you use it leave arms and legs out).

b. If core temperature is less than 86°F (30°C), recommend:
   1. Gastric lavage with warm 107°F (42°C) water—use an ewald gastric tube.
   2. Peritoneal lavage (if no surgical scars on abdomen) using Ringers lactate heated to 107°F (42°C). Run at 8L/hour. After every fourth to fifth liter Ringers use one liter 5% dextrose.

c. If cardiopulmonary bypass is available use for patient:
   1. In cardiac arrest.
   2. With surgical scars on abdomen and severe hypothermia.
   3. With solid frozen extremities.

Emergency Treatment of Frostbite

I. Keep cold until able to rewarm.

II. Rapidly rewarm frozen part in warm 103°F–107°F (39°C–42°C) water. May start in water at 90°F (32°C) and increase to 107°F (42°C) over 15 minutes.

III. After rewarming, *protect* part in bulky dressing. May apply silver sulfadiazine. Pad interdigital areas (use Kerlix rolls and fluffs).
   A. Do *not* break blisters.
   B. Elevate frozen extremities.
   C. Change dressings every 2–3 days.
   D. Continue dressings until all necrotic tissue has sloughed (2½–3 weeks).
IV. Give pain medication as needed.

Selected Readings

MEDICAL REFERENCES

Blair, E., *Clinical Hypothermia*. McGraw-Hill, New York, 1964.

Dripps, R. (Ed.), *The Physiology of Induced Hypythermia*. National Academy of Sciences/National Research Council, Washington, D.C., 1956.

Ferrer, M., *Cold Injury*. Josiah Macy Jr. Foundation, New York, 1954.

Helfferich, C. (Ed.), *Symposia on Arctic Biology and Medicine* (Vol. 1, *The Physiology of Work in Cold and Altitude*). Arctic Aeromedical Laboratory, Ft. Wainwright, Alaska, 1966.

Keatinge, W., *Survival in Cold Water*. Blackwell Scientific, Oxford, 1969.

LeBlanc, J., *Man in the Cold*. Charles Thomas, Springfield, Ill., 1975.

Lomax, P., and E. Schonbaum (Eds.), *Body Temperature: Regulation, Drug Effects and Therapeutic Implications*. Dekker, New York, 1979.

Maclean, D., and D. Emslie-Smith, *Accidental Hypothermia*. Blackwell Scientific, Oxford, 1977.

Popovic, V., and P. Popovic, *Hypothermia in Biology and in Medicine*. Grune and Stratton, New York, 1974.

Pozos, R., and L. Witmers (Eds.), *Proceedings of the Conference on The Nature and Treatment of Hypothermia*. University of Minnesota Press, Minneapolis, Minn., 1982.

Satinoff, E. (Ed.), *Thermoregulation*. Dowden, Hutchinson, and Ross, Stroudsburg, Pa., 1980.

Schilling, C., and P. Story, *Man in the Cold Environment.* Undersea Medical Society, Rockville, Md., 1981.

Schilling, C., M. Werts, and R. Schondelmeir, *The Underwater Handbook: A Guide to Physiology and Performance for the Engineer.* Plenum Press, New York, 1976.

Ward, M., *Mountain Medicine.* Van Nostrand Reinhold, New York, 1975.

Wilkerson, J., *Medicine for Mountaineering.* The Mountaineers, Seattle, Wash., 1975.

SURVIVAL REFERENCES

Bailey, M. and M., *Staying Alive!* David McKay, New York, 1974.

Biggs, D., *Survival Afloat.* David McKay, New York, 1976.

Bridge, R., *The Complete Snow Camper's Guide.* Scribner's, New York, 1973.

Council for National Cooperation in Aquatics, *The New Science of Skin and Scuba Diving.* New Century Publishers, Inc., Piscataway, N.J., 1980.

Dalrymple, B., *Survival in the Outdoors.* Dutton, New York, 1972.

Fear, G., *Surviving the Unexpected Wilderness Emergency.* Survival Education Association, Tacoma, Wash., 1972.

Greenback, A., *The Book of Survival.* Harper and Row, New York, 1967.

Henderson, R., *Sea Sense.* International Marine, Camden, Maine, 1972.

Merrill, B., *The Survival Handbook.* Winchester Press, New York, 1972.

Miller, J., *NOAA Diving Manual.* U.S. Government Printing Office, Washington, D.C., 1979.

Olson, L., *Outdoor Survival Skills.* Brigham Young University Press, Provo, Utah, 1967.

Patterson, C., *Mountain Wilderness Survival.* And/Or Press, Berkeley, Calif., 1979.

Robertson, D., *Sea Survival.* Praeger, New York, 1975.

U.S. Air Force, *Survival!* (U.S.A.F. Manual 64-5). Paladin Enterprises, Boulder, Colo., N.D.

U.S. Army, *Basic Cold Weather Manual* (FM 31-7). Paladin Enterprises, Boulder, Colo., N.D.

Index

171